The Fastest Way to Get

Pregnant Naturally

The
Fastest
Way
to Get
Pregnant
Naturally

The Latest Information on Conceiving a
Healthy Baby on Your Timetable

CHRISTOPHER D. WILLIAMS, M.D.

HYPERION

NEW YORK

Figures 1.3, 3.2, 3.7, 5.2, 5.3, 5.4, 5.5A, 5.5B, 5.7, and 8.3, reprinted with permission from Williams & Williams, Inc., Durham, North Carolina.

Figure 1.5, from American College of Obstetricians and Gynecologists, "Detecting Ovulation," *Planning for Pregnancy, Birth, and Beyond,* 2nd ed. (Washington, DC, 1995). © ACOG. Reprinted with permission.

Figure 1.7, adapted from A. J. Wilcox, C. R. Weinberg, and D. D. Baird, "Timing of Sexual Intercourse in Relation to Ovulation," *New England Journal of Medicine,* 333, no. 23. Copyright © 1995 Massachusetts Medical Society. Reprinted with permission. All rights reserved.

Figures 3.1A, 3.1B, 6.1, 7.7A, and 7.7B, reprinted with permission from *Recommended Dietary Allowances,* 10th ed., © 1989 by the National Academy of Sciences. Courtesy of the National Academy Press, Washington, DC.

Figure 4.1 (identical to Figure 6.3), from B. B. Green, N. S. Weiss, and J. R. Daling, "Risk of Ovulatory Infertility in Relation to Body Weight," *Fertility and Sterility* 50, p. 723. © 1988 Elsevier Science. Reprinted with permission.

Figure 6.2, from J. A. Hodgdon and M. B. Beckett, "Prediction of Percent Body Fat for U.S. Navy Women from Body Circumferences and Height," *NHRC Report* no. 84-29 (1984). Reprinted with permission from Naval Health Research Center.

Figure 10.1, reproduced with the permission of the Alan Guttmacher Institute from J. Bongaarts, "Infertility After Age 30: A False Alarm," Comments, *Family Planning Perspectives,* 14 (2): 77. Copyright © 1982.

Figure 10.2, from Creasy and Resnik, eds., *Maternal Fetal Medicine: Practice and Principles* (Philadelphia: W.B. Saunders), 71. Copyright © 1994. Reproduced with permission from the publisher, Harcourt Health Sciences.

Figure 10.3, reprinted by permission from the American Society for Reproductive Medicine (*Fertility and Sterility,* vol. 46, 989 pp., Gindoff et al., "reproductive potential in older women . . .")

Figure 11.1, from Wilcox, Weinberg, and Baird, "Timing of Sexual Intercourse in Relation to Ovulation," *New England Journal of Medicine,* 333, no. 23. Copyright © 1995 Massachusetts Medical Society. Reprinted with permission. All rights reserved.

Library of Congress Cataloging-in-Publication Data

Williams, Christopher
      The fastest way to get pregnant naturally : the latest information on conceiving a healthy baby on your timetable / Christopher D. Williams.—[2nd ed.]
         p.   cm.
      Includes bibliographical references and index.
      ISBN 1-4013-0870-8
      1. Conception.   2. Fertility, Human.   3. Infertility—Alternative treatment.
I. Title.

   RG133.W555 2006
   618.1'78—dc22   2006043663

Hyperion books are available for special promotions and premiums. For details contact Michael Rentas, Assistant Director, Inventory Operations, Hyperion, 77 West 66th Street, 12th floor, New York, New York 10023, or call 212-456-0133.

SECOND EDITION

10 9 8 7 6 5 4 3 2 1

This book is dedicated to my wife and best friend, Kara, my sons, Scott and Justin, and my daughter, Caroline. The four greatest gifts I will ever receive. Also, to my parents, Richie and Mary Ellen, I will never be able to express to you my appreciation for your love and support.

CONTENTS

ACKNOWLEDGMENTS

TO write a book is truly an immense undertaking. Although only my name appears on the front cover, so many people were critical in this book's content and completion. First and foremost, I want to thank my wife, Kara, for giving me the idea for the book, providing the support and understanding necessary to enable me to write it, and creating or formatting many of the figures. A special thanks to a fantastic freelance editor, Deborah Joy Cafiero. I am indebted to everyone at Hyperion, but especially my editors, Miriam Wenger (second edition) and Mary Ellen O'Neill (first edition), who made the process easier and more enjoyable. My appreciation to my literary agent, Barbara Lowenstein, for believing in the concept. Many thanks to Nancy Marshburn, an excellent medical illustrator, and Kristen Healey, a wonderful graphic artist. I want to acknowledge Kelli Hughes, RD, for her efforts to create Appendix B, "Dietary Information for a Sex-Selection Diet." Special recognition to my parents, Dr. Richard Williams and Mary Ellen Williams, who offered valuable encouragement and constructive criticism on the early manuscript. Of course, I want to thank the many patients whose stories are included in this book.

My appreciation to a number of organizations and publications, including: American College of Obstetricians and Gynecologists, New England Journal of Medicine, National Academy of Sciences/National Academy Press, Elsevier Science, American Society for Reproductive Medicine, W. B. Saunders/Harcourt Health Sciences, Alan Guttmacher Institute, and the Naval Health Research Center. There were many people who made significant contributions merely through simple advice or referrals to other sources. My thanks to Rudy Abramson, Carol Krucoff, Tracy Maxwell, Nancy Cappelman, Dr. James Hogdgon, and Dr. Anthony Hackney. My sincerest apologies to anyone I may have left out.

A final acknowledgment to those people in my professional life who served as role models during my medical training. My sincere appreciation to: Dr. Marc Fritz, Dr. William Meyer, Dr. Bruce Lessey, Dr. Ania Kowalik, Dr. John Boggess, Dr. Paul Marshburn, Dr. Wallace Nunley, Dr. Ronald Wade, Dr. Robert Brame, Dr. Bruce Bateman, and Dr. Siva Thiagarajah—all teachers, mentors, and friends.

AUTHOR'S NOTE

THE information and advice in this book is for educational purposes only. It is intended as a complement to, not a substitute for, the advice of your own physician, with whom you should consult about your individual needs. I recommend that every couple, regardless of medical history, see a doctor for a preconceptional counseling visit prior to attempting to get pregnant. Reading this book prior to the preconceptional visit with your own doctor will be beneficial. Always consult your doctor before starting any treatment or diet. The author and publisher will not be liable for any complications, injuries, or other medical problems arising from or in connection with the use of or reliance upon any information in this book.

The names of the patients included in this book have been changed to ensure anonymity.

INTRODUCTION

WHY do millions of ordinary couples need a guide to getting pregnant? As we begin the twenty-first century, conception for the ordinary couple is a much more complex process than it used to be. It's no longer acceptable to just stop a birth-control method and wait to see what happens. Over two-thirds of all American couples have dual careers, and because of their professional responsibilities they have a preferred timetable for pregnancy. Once couples start trying to become pregnant, it cannot happen fast enough. In addition, many experts now recognize the vital importance of proper diet, weight, exercise, social habits, medical care, and many other factors *before* getting pregnant in order to maximize the health of the baby. This is referred to as preconceptional care.

As an infertility specialist, I spend much of my day with infertile couples discussing conception and pregnancy. When my wife and I decided to try to get pregnant, it became apparent to me how complicated conceiving has become for the "normal" fertile couple. I realized that it is not just infertile couples who need advice. It also became clear that our experience getting pregnant is a very common one. At the same time we were planning our pregnancy, many of our friends and family members had also reached the point in their lives where they wanted to get pregnant. It quickly became apparent that all these healthy couples shared many of the same questions and concerns.

My wife, Kara, a modern woman with a master's degree in computer systems, wanted to learn more about conception so she could conceive as quickly as possible once we started "trying." She also had many questions about what needed to be done preconceptionally to maximize her and the baby's health. Being very independent, she didn't want to ask me all her questions. One Saturday she went to the bookstore to purchase a reference book on how to conceive a healthy baby quickly. Although there were dozens of books on pregnancy and infertility, she could not find a single one written for the "normal," presumably fertile couple about conceiving a healthy baby on your timetable. That was when the idea arose to write this book.

Simple lifestyle choices such as what you eat, how much alcohol or caffeine you drink, your weight, your level of exercise, whether or not you smoke, and the timing of sexual intercourse (among many others) can strongly influence the length of time required to become pregnant. Over 90 percent of couples are fertile, but that doesn't mean you can't enhance your chances of getting pregnant faster or do things to maximize your baby's health. In the last few years home urinary-ovulation-prediction kits have become very popular, evidence of the strong desire of couples to use the latest technology to speed up the process of getting pregnant. Women are looking for the most up-to-date information and advice to allow them to better control their own conception. *The Fastest Way to Get Pregnant Naturally* fulfills all the modern couple's needs with the most recent information and specific recommendations to maximize fertility. And most of the recommendations in this book are easy to implement and don't require a trip to the doctor. The use of the word *Naturally* in the title shouldn't suggest that I don't support technology or appropriate medical interventions when needed. I merely wanted to emphasize the book's focus on ordinary, presumably fertile couples. If you are infertile or require special medical evaluations or treatments before or during pregnancy, then this is not the book for you.

Even if a couple is perfectly healthy and fertile, I recommend that they schedule a preconceptional visit with their family doctor or obstetrician/gynecologist before getting pregnant. No one disputes that this is a fantastic idea for many reasons, but in reality very few couples actually see their physician prior to the pregnancy. Even if they do go, couples still don't know what questions they should be asking or what testing they should request. Because preconceptional care is a relatively new concept and recommendations are being expanded rapidly, many physicians are not aware of all the important aspects to consider. Additionally, as you can see by the length of this book, there's no way you could cover everything in one visit. *The Fastest Way to Get Pregnant Naturally* will help you identify the most important concerns and assure you that your physician is offering the most recent preconceptional recommendations and, in some cases, testing.

For any couple who wants to control the timing and improve the outcome of their pregnancy, this book will give them the preconceptional knowledge to help achieve that goal. *The Fastest Way to Get Pregnant Naturally* will show you ways to help conceive more rapidly, maximize your chances of conceiving a healthy baby, and lower your risk of miscarriage. Simply put, the recommendations offered in these pages will allow ordinary couples to have the healthiest baby as quickly as possible. So read on, enjoy yourselves, and good luck!

The Fastest Way to Get

Pregnant Naturally

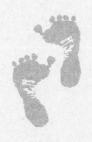

1

The Basics

What a stupendous, what an incomprehensible
machine is [the human body]!

—*Thomas Jefferson, 1786*

YOU'RE about to start learning about your own body.
You will probably read things you never heard of before, and
hopefully you will discover the answers to many of your questions. Getting pregnant quickly, and bearing a healthy child,
can be facilitated by a sound understanding of many different
aspects of your body and how they relate to reproduction.
There is a significant amount of misunderstanding about female anatomy, the menstrual cycle, and ovulation—and how
these reproductive functions interact with a woman's lifestyle
and overall health. Many people also harbor misconceptions,
usually centering on ways to optimize sperm production and
function, about the man's role in reproduction.

The purpose of this chapter is to review the anatomy and
basic physiology of male and female reproduction to lay the
groundwork for the important information found in the chapters that follow. I have written this chapter in very basic terms,

to allow readers to follow along even if they have had no exposure to these ideas since high school "sex education."

FEMALE REPRODUCTIVE ANATOMY

The vagina, uterus, Fallopian tubes, and ovaries are the key anatomical components of the female reproductive system. Together with the brain, they play a vital role in the process of getting pregnant.

The Vagina

The vagina is much more than merely a conduit for sexual intercourse. Few women understand the importance of maintaining the normal bacterial environment of the vagina to

Figure 1.1

FEMALE REPRODUCTIVE ANATOMY

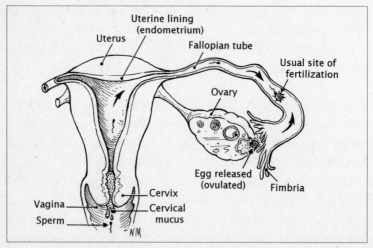

maximize fertility. Avoiding certain practices, such as douching, may help prevent changes in the normal bacterial balance of the vagina that lead to inflammation and infections, and can improve your reproductive health. If you can recognize inflammation and infections of the vagina and make sure you get appropriate treatment promptly, you can help prevent miscarriages, possibly reduce your risk for pelvic inflammatory disease and ectopic pregnancy, and potentially shorten the time required to conceive.

The vagina allows menstrual blood to leave the uterus. It also provides a passage for the penis to deposit sperm as close as possible to the uterus. All skin and mucosal surfaces of our body normally have bacteria that live along the surface, and the vagina is no different. There are many types of "benign" bacteria that live in the vagina, but the predominant one is called *Lactobacillus acidophilus*. These bacteria create an ecosystem in the vagina where the healthy bacteria keep unhealthy bacteria or fungi from invading. A yeast infection is a classic example of a shift in the normal microbial balance; the yeast grow rapidly, resulting in irritation to the vagina's skin surface and causing vaginal discharge. The *Lactobacillus*, along with some other normal bacteria, keep the vagina acidic, with a pH of approximately 4 (any pH below 7 is acidic). Most of the time the normal bacteria and the acidic environment effectively keep other organisms from invading the vagina or overgrowing.

Vaginal douching has little, if any, effect on vaginal pH, but it may disrupt the normal balance of organisms in the vagina. *In some groups of women, douching has been shown to double the risk of developing an infection called bacterial vaginosis*, which results from an overgrowth of abnormal bacteria in the vagina. Although often asymptomatic, bacterial vaginosis can increase the risk for miscarriage, ectopic pregnancy, and pelvic inflammatory disease, and may also lead to a delay in conception (discussed further in Chapter 2). Many women douche after their menses, but this is not necessary, as the vagina is self-cleaning. *For maximum fertility, it's better not to douche and simply let the vagina take care of itself.*

The Uterus and Cervix

People think of the cervix and uterus as two separate organs, but the cervix is actually a part of the uterus. The cervix is the lower portion of the uterus and protrudes down into the uppermost end of the vagina. When your doctor takes a Pap smear, he or she is examining your cervix. If you are comfortable with self-examination, you can feel your own cervix by placing one or two fingers into your vagina and locating a knob of tissue all the way at the end. The cervix is about as firm as the end of your nose. You should feel a small dimple in the center of the cervix—this is the opening to the cervical canal.

This cervical opening, or canal, allows the sperm to travel from the vagina into the uterus. The cervix is the doorway for the sperm to enter the uterus and for menstrual blood to leave the uterus. The cervix also is the part of the uterus that must dilate to allow delivery of the baby during labor.

Within the cervical canal are mucous glands. Cervical mucus, which makes up the majority of the fluid from the vagina, changes its consistency during the menstrual cycle. Many women notice that in the first half of their cycle the mucus goes from a minimal amount of thick, sticky substance to a plentiful, thin, watery, stretchy fluid that feels slippery. Estrogen levels are rising in the first half of the menstrual cycle and peak by midcycle. The thin, slippery mucus is much easier for the sperm to swim through, so it gets maximally produced at the most fertile time of the month, around the time of ovulation. The cervix also has "crypts," or deep folds, where the sperm can pool after ejaculation. The sperm may stay there for as long as two to three days after intercourse, increasing the chances of fertilization. I will consider these changes in cervical mucus for ovulation prediction in more detail in Chapter 5.

The uterus, or womb, is one of the hardest-working tissues in the body. Normally the size of a fist, the uterus lies in the pelvis behind the bladder and in front of the rectum. Not only does the uterus hold the baby during pregnancy, but it also is constantly forming or shedding its inner lining when a woman is not pregnant. This lining is called the endometrium, and it is vital to the implantation and growth of the fertilized egg.

Fallopian Tubes

The two Fallopian tubes run from the uterus to the ovaries. The Fallopian tubes are much more than simple conduits for the sperm to reach the ovaries. They contain fingerlike projections at their ends, called fimbria, which extend out across the surface of the ovary and are able to pick up the egg and bring it into the tube. Once the egg is inside the Fallopian tube, tiny projections called cilia sweep the egg along the inside of the tube and into the uterus. The Fallopian tube also contracts in muscular waves that help push the egg toward the uterus. *When an egg is fertilized by a sperm, it usually takes place in the Fallopian tube.* The muscular contractions and cilia of the Fallopian tube then sweep the fertilized egg into the uterus, where implantation normally occurs.

Selena, 34, recently had an embryo, or very early developing pregnancy, implant in her left Fallopian tube instead of in her uterus. This misplaced location of a pregnancy is referred to as an ectopic pregnancy. Surgical removal of Selena's left tube was required. Several years earlier her right ovary had been removed because of a benign ovarian tumor. Selena wanted to know whether she could still get pregnant now that she didn't have a Fallopian tube and ovary on the same side.

I explained to her that only one functional tube is necessary to become pregnant. A woman with Selena's problem—with one Fallopian tube and one ovary on opposite sides—can still become pregnant. After ovulation, the egg can be picked up by the Fallopian tube on the opposite side, although it's significantly less efficient than having the tube on the same side. Women with Selena's problem can get pregnant, but it would be expected to take much longer than the average time.

The Ovaries

Two ovaries lie behind the uterus, adjacent to the Fallopian tubes. The ovaries are glands; that is, they secrete hormones, mainly estrogen and progesterone. The ovaries also hold a woman's eggs. When she starts getting her menstrual cycle, an adolescent female has about 400,000 eggs. By the time a woman goes through menopause, her eggs will be all gone. Women don't grow more eggs or replace them in adulthood, the way men do sperm.

The quality of the eggs is most strongly correlated with the age of the woman. As a woman ages so do her ovaries, and the ability for the eggs to be fertilized, implant into the uterus, and grow is progressively compromised. Diminished egg quality is the main reason why older women have higher rates of infertility and miscarriage. I will discuss the relationship between age and fertility in detail in Chapters 10 and 12.

Once ovulated, that is, once it has left the ovary, the egg survives for only 12 to 24 hours. This leaves a narrow window of opportunity for fertilization to occur. To get pregnant as fast as possible, it's essential to pinpoint the exact day of ovulation. Chapter 5 is devoted entirely to this important subject.

The Brain

The brain is the conductor of the orchestra of the menstrual cycle. Two main areas of the brain—the hypothalamus and the pituitary—release the hormones that control the menstrual cycle. Follicle stimulating hormone (FSH) and luteinizing hormone (LH) are the primary menstrual hormones released by the brain. FSH serves mainly to stimulate growth of the ovarian "follicle," a small cyst in the ovary that holds the egg inside, whereas LH is the hormone that stimulates the egg to be released from the ovary. Home ovulation-prediction kits test for the presence of LH.

The brain can be influenced by many outside stimuli, leading to irregularities in the menstrual cycle and decreased fertility. Stress, illness, poor nutrition, excessive exercise, extremes of weight, and many other external factors commonly affect menstrual regularity. I'll review many of these influences in subsequent chapters.

MALE ANATOMY AND REPRODUCTIVE FUNCTION

Society is biased in its perspective on fertility. Almost uniformly, people assume that when a couple is having problems getting pregnant, those problems are probably caused by the female partner. In reality, the male partner is directly responsible for the delay in conception in at least 40 percent of cases and is a significant contributor to infertility 60 percent of the time. For this reason, Chapter 8 is devoted specifically to what

Figure 1.2
THE MALE REPRODUCTIVE ANATOMY

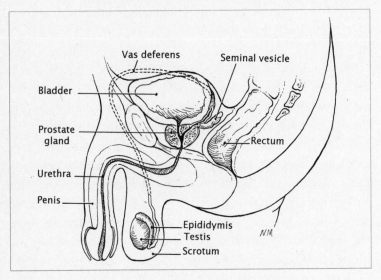

a man can do to maximize a couple's chance of conceiving a healthy baby as quickly as possible. For now, I'll review the basic anatomy and reproductive function of the male partner to help you understand the recommendations that follow in subsequent chapters.

The Penis

The main role of the penis is to deposit sperm as close as possible to a woman's cervix. The penis also allows the urine from the bladder to drain through the urethra, a tube that runs through the center of the penis. When a man ejaculates, or has an orgasm, his semen moves into the urethra, and muscular contractions force the semen out the end of the penis. These rhythmic involuntary contractions are what make up the sensation of orgasm for the male. Although male orgasm is necessary for pregnancy to occur, female orgasm is not.

The Testicles

Sperm are produced in the testicles. The testicles produce millions of sperm each day. Greater than 20 million sperm per milliliter of semen ejaculated is considered a normal sperm count, with the average sperm count around 60 million per milliliter. This may seem like a lot of sperm, but consider how small the microscopic egg is in the expanse of a woman's ovary, Fallopian tube, and uterus. Having such an enormous number of sperm to travel through the woman's reproductive tract, especially since the sperm can stay in the cervical crypts for days before moving into the uterus, greatly increases the chance that one sperm will encounter the egg at just the right moment for fertilization.

The testicles hang in a sac, called the scrotum, outside the body. Muscles inside the scrotum contract and relax, raising and lowering the testicles in relation to the body. This is because the optimal temperature for sperm production is lower than normal core body temperature (98.6 degrees Fahrenheit). It has long been suspected that certain types of clothing or activities may lead to higher testicular temperatures, lower sperm counts, and reduced fertility for the man. Recent studies—including ones that examine the effects of boxers versus briefs—indicate that this concern has been overstated (see Chapter 8).

Why does it take only one egg but at least 20 million sperm in order to become pregnant? Because men never ask for directions.

Figure 1.3

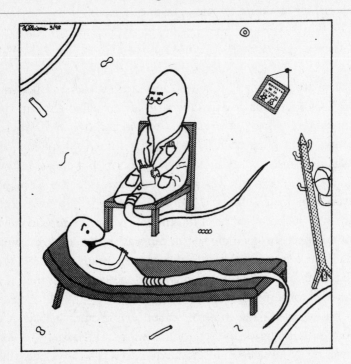

You just never know doc... Any day could be the day. And then, competing with 50 million other guys for just one egg! The stress is killing me!

It takes about 72 days for a sperm to mature and be available for ejaculation. The prolonged time required for maturation of the sperm means that *any factor influencing sperm production wouldn't have an impact on the sperm count until about three months later.* Many common outside influences can affect sperm production, including tobacco and alcohol use, viral illnesses such as the common cold or flu, physical trauma, temperature, frequency of intercourse, some medications, and "recreational" drugs.

Semen contains the sperm and surrounding fluid, predominantly the product of secretions from the seminal vesicles and the prostate gland. These two glands deposit fluid at the time of orgasm that mixes with the sperm. Because these secretions make up almost the entire volume of the semen, merely looking at how much semen is ejaculated is not a good indicator of whether you have a high or low sperm count.

PREGNANCY AND THE MONTHLY CYCLE

The menstrual cycle is a continual process of hormonal changes that lead to the preparation of the uterine lining, ovulation, and then shedding of the lining if pregnancy doesn't take place. Every day of the menstrual cycle brings important events in the ovaries and the uterine lining. Each month, an egg must be selected and then stimulated to become mature, and the uterine lining must be prepared in case a fertilized egg (embryo) arrives to implant and grow.

The menstrual cycle is commonly called the "monthly cycle" because it lasts approximately one month in most women. Some people believe the menstrual cycles should follow the months of the calendar. However, the menstrual cycle will not occur on the same day each month, since calendar months are not equal in length, and, because the body is not a clock, each woman has some variability between cycles.

Tyla, 22, came to see me because she had been having two menstrual periods each month for the last four months. She brought a few menstrual calendars with her to illustrate the problem. When I examined the calendars I found that her menstrual cycles were about 24 days. The cycles began in the first few days of the month and then returned again the last

Figure 1.4
VARIATIONS IN THE MENSTRUAL CYCLE

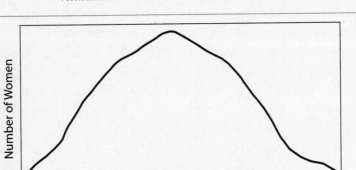

The exact middle of the curve falls on 28 days. This is the average cycle length, but the vast majority of women do not have cycles that are 28 days in length.

few days of the same month. I reassured her that 24-day menstrual cycles are considered normal and she need not be concerned.

You can count the days in your menstrual cycle by assigning the first day of menstrual bleeding as cycle day 1. The average female cycle length is about 28 days. More accurately, the average menstrual cycle length changes throughout life and is closer to 30 days when a woman is 20 years old and 26 days on average when a woman approaches menopause around age 50. Only a minority of women actually have a 28-day cycle, while any cycle length between 24 and 35 days is considered normal. A woman's body varies from month to month, and few women have exactly the same number of days in each of their menstrual cycles.

Figure 1.5
IMPORTANT ASPECTS OF THE MENSTRUAL CYCLE

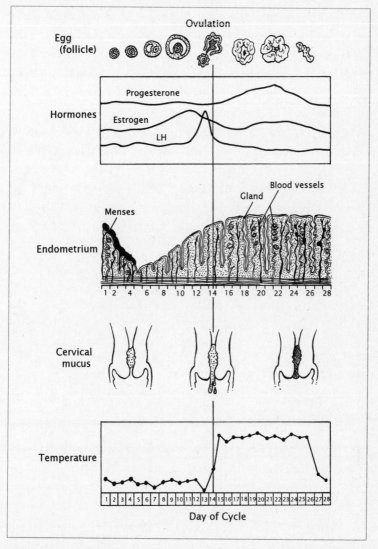

Reprinted with permission from the American College of Obstetricians and Gynecologists, *Planning for Pregnancy, Birth, and Beyond*, 2nd ed. (Washington, D.C. 1995). ©ACOG.

Ovulation

From the woman's perspective, ovulation, or the release of the egg from the ovary, is usually the single most important factor in becoming pregnant as quickly as possible. Understanding the process of ovulation is vital in order to time your intercourse appropriately and maximize your chances of getting pregnant each month. Chapter 5 is dedicated to this important subject; therefore, we will only introduce the topic in this section.

During the first half of the menstrual cycle, a woman's body produces increasing amounts of estrogen and follicle stimulating hormone (FSH). FSH stimulates the growth of the egg to be released (ovulated) that month, while estrogen causes the uterus to prepare for possible pregnancy by growing a thick (endometrial) lining. The choice of which ovary will release

Figure 1.6

HORMONAL CHANGES DURING A
28-DAY MENSTRUAL CYCLE

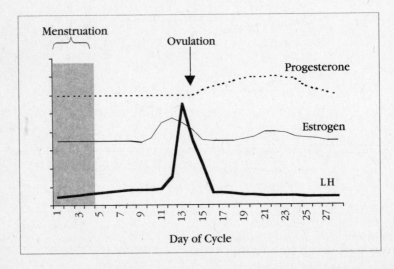

the egg in any given cycle is random. Ovulation occurs around the middle of each menstrual cycle, usually about 14 days before a woman's menstrual cycle (bleeding) begins.

A woman with the average cycle length, 28 days, will probably ovulate on cycle day 14. However, because women with normal menstrual cycles can have cycle lengths anywhere between 24 and 35 days, this simple "14-day rule" doesn't generate a precise enough prediction to allow you to time your intercourse accurately. *Even if you timed the length of your previous menstrual cycle, your body is not a clock and your cycle may not be exactly the same length from month to month.* That's why this book stresses reliable ovulation-prediction methods as a vital component to conceiving as rapidly as possible. When rising estrogen levels in the bloodstream reach their peak, this triggers the brain to release a hormone called luteinizing hormone (LH), which signals the ovary to release the egg. The brain releases the LH into the bloodstream. When the LH in the bloodstream reaches the ovary, ovulation will occur about 36 hours later. LH is important to remember because it is the hormone measured by the home ovulation-prediction kits. These kits can be purchased over the counter in any pharmacy and are extremely popular. (The urinary kits, and other methods for ovulation prediction, are discussed in great detail in Chapter 5.)

The remaining empty follicle, from which the egg was released, then re-forms into a fluid-filled sac, or cyst, known as the corpus luteum. It is the corpus luteum that produces the hormone progesterone following ovulation. Progesterone dominates the second half of the menstrual cycle, while levels of estrogen wane. Progesterone causes the lining of the uterus to make the final preparations necessary for the implantation and growth of the early pregnancy in the uterus. Rising levels of progesterone cause a woman's core body temperature to rise significantly. This temperature change serves as the basis for the basal body temperature (BBT) method of predicting ovulation.

Fertilization and Implantation

Once sperm have entered the vagina, they must swim up through the cervix, through the uterus, and into the Fallopian tubes to find the released egg. The union of sperm and egg is called fertilization. *Sperm have the best success rate of fertilizing the egg for up to 48 to 72 hours (two to three days) following intercourse. The egg, however, can survive for no more than 12 to 24 hours.* This creates a narrow window of opportunity for the sperm and egg to unite. When the egg is fertilized by a sperm an embryo is formed, and conception has taken place. The embryo is the earliest stage of a developing baby.

Six or seven days after ovulation, the embryo implants in the lining of the uterus. Within a few days a hormone called human chorionic gonadotropin (hCG) is made by the newly implanted embryo. This hCG is the hormone measured by the home pregnancy test kits that are sold in all drugstores.

Even though the embryo implants within seven days after ovulation, not enough hCG is produced for the urinary pregnancy test to become positive until three to seven days after implantation. For this reason, it takes at least 10 days after fertilization, but more commonly 14 days, before a urinary pregnancy test will indicate a positive result. This means that if you know (or suspect) the day you conceived, you shouldn't perform a urine pregnancy test until 10 to 14 days later—or better yet, simply wait 14 days, because if you test your urine and have a negative result 10 days after conception you will need to repeat the test four days later anyway. If you don't know when in the cycle you may have conceived, wait until you are

Figure 1.7
PROBABILITY OF CONCEPTION ON SPECIFIC DAYS
NEAR THE DAY OF OVULATION

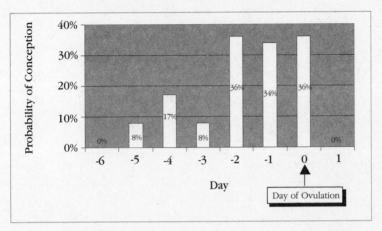

The bars represent probabilities calculated from data on 129 menstrual cycles in which sexual intercourse was recorded to have occurred on only a *single* day during the six-day interval ending on the day of ovulation (day 0). Note that intercourse one day after ovulation results in no pregnancies, and a single episode of intercourse the day of ovulation and up to two days before ovulation have an equal chance of conception—about 35 percent.

(Adapted with permission from: A.J. Wilcox, C.R. Weinberg, and D.D. Baird, "Timing of Sexual Intercourse in Relation to Ovulation." *The New England Journal of Medicine*, 333, no. 23 (1995): 1519. Copyright © 1995, Massachusetts Medical Society. All rights reserved.)

a few days late for your menstrual period and then perform a home pregnancy test. The pregnancy tests that can be purchased at a pharmacy use the same technologies as the test kits found in your doctor's office, so you don't need to spend the extra time getting a urinary pregnancy test from your physician.

Figure 1.8

FERTILIZATION

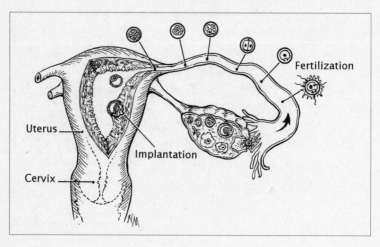

Figure 1.9

KEY HORMONES OF THE MENSTRUAL CYCLE,
OVULATION, AND PREGNANCY

Estrogen—The hormone that rises continuously during the first two weeks of the menstrual cycle. Estrogen promotes the growth of a thick uterine lining, or endometrium. Estrogen also causes changes in the character and amount of cervical mucus.

Progesterone—The hormone that is produced during the second half of the menstrual cycle. Progesterone prepares the uterus to allow the fertilized egg to implant and grow. If pregnancy doesn't occur, progesterone levels drop and the uterus sheds its lining, resulting in menstrual bleeding.

Luteinizing Hormone (LH)—The hormone released from the brain that is responsible for release of the egg from the ovary, or ovulation. Ovulation usually occurs about 36 hours after the rise in LH. Home ovulation-prediction kits test for elevated levels of LH.

Human Chorionic Gonadotropin (hCG)—The hormone produced by the developing embryo. Home pregnancy tests detect the presence of hCG.

At this point you should have all the information necessary to understand the chapters that follow. My hope is that you learned a few things without getting too bored with the details. In many of the subsequent chapters, I will expand upon the information mentioned in this chapter. Now let's get you started preparing to conceive a healthy baby as quickly as possible.

2

Am I Fertile?

How do I know if I can get pregnant?

—*Tricia, 31*

EVERY couple wonders at one time or another: how do we know if we're fertile? Tricia's question expresses what all women would like to know before they start the exciting, but frequently nerve-racking, process of conceiving. Many couples are looking for reassurance that they won't run into problems getting pregnant.

This chapter reviews the most common issues that affect women in their reproductive years. Because this is a book for presumably fertile couples, I was asked why I included a chapter on gynecologic problems that may have a negative impact on fertility. The fact is, most fertile women will have at least one of the concerns I address in this chapter. But, if you recognize yourself in any of these descriptions, don't be alarmed—*the vast majority of women with one or more of these conditions will conceive without difficulty.* The purpose of this chapter is not to alarm, but rather to educate, inform, and in nearly all cases reassure. Most of the time there are ways to minimize the impact of these conditions on your fertility; here I will reveal the often simple methods to help you get pregnant as fast as possible.

Nearly all couples are fertile and should be optimistic about their chances of conceiving a healthy baby in a rapid time frame. *Only about one in ten couples will not succeed in becoming pregnant within one year of trying.* This 90 percent success rate does not apply only to couples with no past or present medical problems. On the contrary, the data used to measure this success rate comes from a cross section of all types of couples. Additionally, this research was done with couples who did not use any of the technology available today—such as ovulation-prediction test kits and computerized, handheld fertility monitors—and who had no knowledge of the fertility-enhancing recommendations and information found in this book. There is every reason to believe that your conception could be *even more rapid* if you apply recent preconceptual recommendations and the latest technology available for home use.

The male partner is equally important in the process of conceiving a healthy baby rapidly, and Chapter 8 is dedicated to male fertility issues. For this reason I will focus my attention on women's issues in this chapter. Keep in mind that this book is intended for average, presumably fertile couples. Although this chapter surveys many common gynecologic concerns that can impact fertility, it is by no means a comprehensive review or treatment guide for these problems.

FIBROIDS

Ileana, 34, came to see me because she was feeling increasing pelvic pressure over the last few months. She also noticed her pants becoming tighter and realized she was wearing her belt one or two notches wider than usual. Ileana was a petite woman, standing five feet two inches tall and weighing about 100 pounds and hadn't gained a single pound, so she could not attribute her symptoms to weight gain. Her menstrual periods had not changed, and she was experiencing no abdominal pain. I performed a physical exam and made the diagnosis of a fibroid uterus.

Fibroid tumors, also referred to as fibroids, uterine leiomyomata, or uterine myomas, are benign growths of smooth muscle tissue in the uterus. They are extremely common, affecting one in five (20 percent) of Caucasian women and up to one in three African-American women. Clearly, fibroids do not usually cause fertility problems—otherwise one-fifth of the Caucasian population and one-third of the African-American population would be infertile from fibroids alone! In a minority of cases, however, fibroids may interfere with the appropriate implantation and early growth of a pregnancy, resulting in decreased fertility or miscarriage.

In many women fibroids occur randomly, but sometimes they appear to run in families. Fibroids that affect reproduction are most common in older reproductive-age women (35 to 45), simply because older women's bodies have had more time to create the large fibroids that can affect fertility.

A fibroid arises from the abnormal growth of a single smooth muscle cell in the wall of the uterus. For reasons largely unknown, the cell receives the wrong growth signals and continues to divide and multiply long after it should have stopped. Over time, the single cell grows into a small ball and may become quite large. During my ob/gyn residency I took care of a patient who allowed a fibroid to grow to the size of a soccer ball before her family talked her into surgical removal.

Common Symptoms of Fibroids

Usually fibroids cause no symptoms, and they are often found during a woman's yearly gynecological exam. The most common symptom of fibroids is heavy, prolonged, and/or painful menstrual periods. However, prolonged or heavy menses with or without pain can indicate a number of possible problems, not just fibroids. Other less common symptoms of fibroids include a feeling of abdominal pressure, abdominal distension (a woman might notice her pants growing tighter despite no weight gain), recurrent miscarriage, infertility, uterine pain even when a woman isn't premenstrual or menstrual, increased urgency or frequency of urination, and loss of bladder control. Once again, most women with fibroids have no significant symptoms.

Location of Fibroids

There are three general locations for fibroids in the uterus (see Figure 2.1). The fibroid can lie within the cavity of the uterus, inside the wall of the uterus, or on the external surface of the uterus. If you have been diagnosed with fibroids but you have no symptoms, this usually indicates that the fibroid(s) is deep within the wall of your uterus or at the external surface of the uterus. The location of the fibroid appears to be the most important factor in whether or not it causes any symptoms or has an adverse effect on reproduction. Fibroids within the wall or at the external surface of the uterus usually will not significantly affect the lining of the uterus (the endometrium), where the pregnancy grows and the tissue is shed during menstrual periods.

The fibroids that grow either in the uterine cavity or inside the wall of the uterus, and become large enough to deform or

Figure 2.1
LOCATION OF FIBROIDS

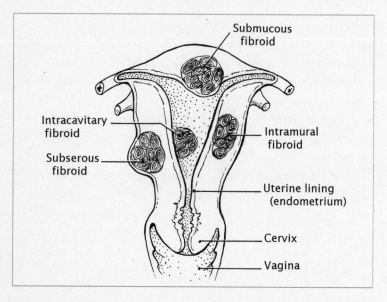

Uterine fibroids can grow within the uterus, inside the uterine wall, or on the outside of the uterus.

distort the uterine cavity and the endometrium, appear to have the highest risk for causing menstrual disturbances, miscarriage, and decreased fertility. The endometrium and uterine cavity may not work normally, leading to bleeding problems, difficulty in implantation, and sometimes miscarriage.

You should know, however, that the link between fibroids and adverse reproductive outcomes is controversial. The American College of Obstetricians and Gynecologists issued a "Technical Bulletin" in 1994 that reviewed fibroids and stated, "there [are] no controlled data to support a causal association between

uterine leiomyomata [fibroids] and adverse reproductive outcomes . . . infertility secondary to leiomyomata is probably
rare." Because fibroids are so common, I wouldn't be in a hurry
to ascribe a couple's infertility or miscarriages to fibroids.

Michelle, 27, came to see me because, as she said, "I'm having ter-
rible cramping and heavy bleeding each month and it seems to be
getting worse." She told me that she and her husband were thinking about starting their family in a year or so. During her physical
exam I found multiple fibroids in her uterus. Because she didn't
want to get pregnant for at least a year, we decided to try oral contraceptives to reduce her bleeding and cramping each month.

Michelle returned three months later for a follow-up appointment and reexamination. Her fibroids had not grown,
and her menstrual periods had normalized on the birth-control
pill. Michelle made plans to stop her birth-control pills in nine
months and then start trying to get pregnant.

Michelle asked if she needed to do anything else about the
fibroids before attempting to conceive. I told her what I tell
almost all my patients with fibroids: unless she had discomfort,
abdominal pressure, abnormal bleeding unresponsive to medication, unless the fibroids had grown rapidly (which is un-
characteristic of fibroids), or, finally, unless the fibroids were
suspected to be the cause of repetitive miscarriages or prolonged infertility, I suggested no other medical or surgical treatment be taken before attempting to conceive.

Four months after stopping her birth-control pills, I received
a phone call from Michelle announcing that she was pregnant.
The pregnancy progressed normally, and her son, Jeremy, was
born one week prior to his due date.

Treatment for Fibroids

The heavy bleeding and severe cramping that are the most common symptoms of fibroids are usually responsive to medications such as birth-control pills and nonsteroidal anti-inflammatory agents (for example, ibuprofen or naproxen sodium). If your symptoms do not resolve with medications, your doctor will often refer you for an ultrasound, or a new ultrasound technique called sonohysterography or hydrosonography. These tests will confirm the existence of fibroids, measure the size of the fibroid(s), and determine its location within the uterus. Unless your symptoms are untreatable or refractory to medical treatment, your fibroids are very large, or you have a history of adverse reproductive outcomes—such as recurrent miscarriage or infertility—you would probably not need surgery to remove the fibroids. Very few women meet the criteria necessary to require special treatment for fibroids before attempting to conceive on their own. *Usually, no special testing or treatments are needed if you are experiencing no symptoms from your fibroids and want to try to conceive.*

Some physicians have recommended a diet for women that may be able to suppress the growth of existing fibroids and prevent the formation of new ones. I will discuss the relationship between diet and fibroids in more detail in Chapter 7.

When fibroids cause problems and conservative treatment measures are not effective, then surgery is often suggested. In order to retain your fertility you will need to make sure that you receive a myomectomy, not a hysterectomy. In a myomectomy the fibroids are removed but the uterus is left in place. The myomectomy is usually done through an incision in your abdomen, but sometimes can be performed through laparoscopic surgery, using a small camera inserted through the navel, or hysteroscopic surgery, with a small camera placed through the vagina and into the uterus.

Ileana, who was introduced at the beginning of this chapter, had pressure symptoms from her fibroid. I performed an ultrasound that showed she had one mango-size fibroid on the outer surface of the top of her uterus. This fibroid undoubtedly would not have altered her fertility in any way, because it was well away from the inner cavity of the uterus. Ileana was engaged to be married, so she had not started her family yet. She wanted to get rid of the pressure symptoms, but she also needed to preserve her fertility. Because there is no medication that can permanently shrink fibroids, I suggested she undergo a myomectomy. I removed the fibroid by an abdominal myomectomy a few months later without complication. When she returned for her postoperative visit she told me, "I feel like I'm back to normal." Ileana has not attempted to conceive yet, but I'm certain that the surgery will have little or no impact on her fertility.

If you need surgery for fibroids, don't worry. Fertility after a myomectomy is usually excellent. If your doctor tells you that a myomectomy cannot be done and that you need a hysterectomy, seek a second opinion! It is a very rare fibroid uterus on which a skilled gynecologic surgeon cannot successfully perform a myomectomy. If your obstetrician/gynecologist doesn't believe that a myomectomy can be performed successfully, you should ask for a referral to a specialist called a *reproductive endocrinologist* for a second opinion.

ENDOMETRIOSIS

Endometriosis describes the presence of normal endometrial tissue (the uterine lining) outside of the uterus. Usually this tissue stays in the pelvis, but in some cases it can be found outside the pelvic cavity. The actual incidence of endometriosis is uncertain, but it is estimated at 2 to 5 percent of the female population. There is a familial predisposition, and women who have a mother or sister with endometriosis have as much as a tenfold increased risk of getting it themselves.

Researchers have explored a number of theories about why endometriosis occurs, but the most commonly accepted explanation is called "retrograde menstruation." In this theory, menstrual flow not only comes down through the cervix and out the vagina during the menstrual period as it's supposed to do, but also goes the opposite direction—up through the Fallopian tubes and out into the pelvis. Some of the fragments of endometrial lining implant on the surface of pelvic organs—such as the ovaries, bladder, or external surface of the Fallopian tubes—and continue to grow, resulting in endometriosis. As one of my patients said, "It's when the lining of the uterus grows in the wrong place."

These abnormally placed endometrial fragments respond to the hormonal cycle just like the normal endometrium inside the uterus. Because of this, endometriosis and normal endometrium undergo similar growth and bleeding phases during the cycle. The body's defenses recognize the presence of endometriosis as abnormal and attack the tissue, resulting in local inflammation and scarring. Because the endometriosis is usually on or close to the ovaries and Fallopian tubes, it is thought that the inflammation can interfere with the ability of the sperm to fertilize the egg, but more research is necessary. In more severe cases, the inflammation and scarring can damage reproductive organs, or the scar tissue can envelop the ovaries or tubes, effectively forming a barrier between the sperm and egg.

Margaret, 30, described her symptoms of endometriosis in the following words: "The pain comes a few days before my period is going to start, peaks just when I start to have my period, and then disappears by about the third day of my period when the bleeding is tapering off." As Margaret emphasizes, women with this condition tend to experience a very clear pattern of discomfort, which predictably follows the menstrual cycle from month to month. The most common symptom of endometriosis is pelvic or back pain that worsens just before and at the beginning of the menstrual period, and then subsides as the period continues. Other symptoms include pain associated with deep thrusting during intercourse, pain with bowel movements (especially around the time of menstrual bleeding), and infertility.

Occurring in as much as 5 percent of the female population, endometriosis is common. It can be associated with infertility, but in many cases it will *not* cause infertility. The presence of a mild case of endometriosis should not be diagnosed as the cause of infertility unless all other reasonable causes have been ruled out. Even if a woman is infertile and has endometriosis, the relationship may be coincidental rather than causative. In addition, because pelvic pain and uncomfortable menstrual periods can arise from a variety of causes, you can't conclude the presence of endometriosis from symptoms alone. Sometimes your physician may be able to feel, or palpate, suspicious areas during the pelvic exam; less commonly, the doctor may recognize areas of possible endometriosis by ultrasound. In nearly all cases, though, the only way to diagnose endometriosis is through surgery, usually laparoscopic. Therefore, many women who have painful menstrual periods are told they may have endometriosis and are treated empirically—meaning, assuming that it is present. Don't panic if your doctor has diagnosed endometriosis. The majority of women who have it will not experience fertility problems, although suppressive medications

Donna, 36, had both a mother and a sister with severe endometriosis. Donna herself had uncomfortable and heavy menstrual periods, and she came to see me requesting a laparoscopy to diagnose and treat what she presumed to be endometriosis. When I conducted the physical exam, everything was normal. I told her that it was quite possible she had endometriosis, but I suggested she consider a conservative medical approach to treatment before considering surgery. We agreed to try to treat her problems with oral contraceptives first. "My periods are much better now" was Donna's comment at her return visit to see me three months later. Because her symptoms had markedly improved, she stayed on the birth-control pills for the next year.

At the age of 37, Donna decided she wanted to get pregnant, and again made an appointment with me to schedule a laparoscopy. "At my age, I don't want to waste a year trying to get pregnant and then have to undergo surgery to get rid of the endometriosis. Why don't we just do the surgery now and my fertility will be maximized right from the start?" Donna made some good points, but I convinced her that even if she had endometriosis, her fertility wouldn't measurably change in the next six months and it would be better for her to try to conceive on her own first, using ovulation-prediction kits (see Chapter 5) to help time intercourse appropriately.

During the sixth month of attempting to conceive, Donna became pregnant. Most interesting to her, though, was what she learned during her baby's delivery. Donna needed a cesarean section, and she told me, "During the c-section my doctor didn't see *any signs* of endometriosis. Can you believe that?"

are often indicated to minimize the condition until you are ready to conceive or between pregnancies.

Treatment for Endometriosis

Endometriosis is a chronic disorder. Even if you treat endometriosis with surgery, removing all visible signs, it is likely that it will return in the future. If you have been diagnosed with endometriosis through surgery, or if your physician suspects endometriosis but thinks surgery is unnecessary, you do have medical options that are very helpful in minimizing the effects of the endometriosis to allow you to maximally preserve your fertility. To maximize your chances to conceive naturally, you and your doctor should discuss the use of suppressive medications until you are ready to try to get pregnant.

My most common recommendation for suppression of chronic endometriosis, especially in patients who wish to preserve their fertility, is to start oral contraceptives. Estrogen is the main stimulus in the growth of endometriosis, whereas progesterone is the main inhibitor of growth. The overall effect of the oral contraceptive is progesterone-like. Progesterone-like effects make the normal endometrium in the uterus thinner and should also make the endometriosis shrink. Additionally, some researchers believe there is less chance of retrograde menstruation, which would further spread the endometriosis. Other effective chronic treatments include Depo-Provera (Upjohn), an intramuscular injection of medroxyprogesterone acetate— again, a progesterone-like medication—every twelve weeks, or daily oral therapy with medroxyprogesterone acetate or other progesterone-like oral medications. Gonadotropin-releasing hormone agonists, the most common being luprolide acetate, or Lupron, can be a very effective short-term treatment of endometriosis, because they effectively shut down nearly all estrogen production. The short-term side effects are the same as those associated with menopause (for example, hot flashes), and these medications also provoke the unfavorable long-term side effects of menopause, notably bone-density loss (osteoporosis). For these reasons gonadotropin-releasing hormone agonists are commonly not employed for more than three to six months, so they're not useful for chronic therapy. Danocrine (Danazol) would be another option, but side effects such as acne, oily skin, unwanted hair growth, weight gain, water retention, and adverse cholesterol changes have made it less popular.

Your diet may also influence the symptoms and progression of endometriosis. There have been a few studies that evaluate the ability of diet to decrease the inflammation and scarring associated with endometriosis. The evidence for altering your diet if you have endometriosis, and what the diet should be, is discussed in Chapter 7.

Even if you have undergone successful surgery to treat endometriosis, I strongly recommend that you either try to become pregnant soon after the surgery or start oral contraceptives or other medical therapy and consider altering your diet to keep the endometriosis at bay until you're ready to start trying to conceive.

INFECTIONS

Bacterial Vaginosis

In Chapter 1, I emphasized the importance of the normal balance of vaginal bacteria. The most common bacteria to overgrow and cause changes in pH and inflammation of the vagina is called *Gardnerella vaginalis*. Overgrowth of *Gardnerella vaginalis* results in an infection of the vagina called bacterial vaginosis (BV). The relationship of BV with miscarriage and preterm labor is now well accepted by the medical community. Associations with ectopic pregnancy and pelvic inflammatory disease have also been demonstrated. I strongly suspect that this infection will be found to play an important role in fertility when appropriately designed studies are performed to examine this question.

Gwynn, 22, gives a common description of BV: "I've had a milky discharge and a strong odor for the last week or two. It's not like the yeast infections I've had in the past, which had a cottage-cheesy discharge and were very itchy." If you think you might have BV, you should make an appointment to see your doctor. This is an easy condition to treat but requires a prescription for antibiotics from your physician.

SEXUALLY TRANSMITTED DISEASES (STDs)

In the 1990s, the HIV epidemic in the United States led to an unparalleled push for public health education for sexually transmitted diseases (STDs). The focus was on "safe sex" to not only prevent the spread of the HIV virus, but also to reduce unwanted pregnancies. What this public campaign did not emphasize is the relationship between STDs and infertility.

The good news is that the vast majority of women with a history of a treated STD will experience no long-term effects from the infection. A minority of women may suffer permanent damage to the reproductive organs from a single infection, but repeat infections are particularly worrisome. Prevention is the most important factor. Although little can be done about a previous infection, future infections are almost always avoidable.

Gonorrhea and Chlamydia

The most common STDs that can affect fertility are gonorrhea (*Neisseria gonorrhea*) and chlamydia (*Chlamydia trachomatis*). These are bacteria that live in the male and female reproductive tracts and are transmitted by sexual intercourse. In the female, the infection begins in the cervix, where it causes inflammation, pain, and often a heavy, purulent (pus) discharge. If left untreated the infection will ascend the female genital tract through the uterus (endometritis), Fallopian tubes (salpingitis), on to the ovaries (oophoritis), and then into the pelvis and abdomen resulting in pelvic inflammatory disease (PID). When the infection spreads beyond the cervix, the symptoms become more severe and often include fever, chills, abdominal pain, nausea and vomiting, and loss of appetite. The key is to treat the infection before it spreads from the cervix. If treated early, the risk of permanent damage to the reproductive organs is much lower. With one episode of PID the risk of permanent infertility is about 10 percent. After the second episode of PID the risk is 25 percent, and after the third episode about half of all infected women will be infertile.

Priscilla, 29, reported that she had a case of chlamydia when she was in college, about ten years earlier. She had unprotected intercourse with a new boyfriend, and within a week she noticed some heavy vaginal discharge. Her doctor examined her and told her that she had gonorrhea or chlamydia and treated her with oral antibiotics for a week.

Priscilla and her husband had started trying to conceive three months before I saw her but had not had any success. I explained that there was no need to do any testing for tubal damage until they had already tried to get pregnant for a reasonable period of time, at least six to nine months. Her risk for infertility from one chlamydial infection of her cervix was probably significantly less than 10 percent, assuming the infection was localized to her cervix and never spread up into her uterus and Fallopian tubes to become PID.

She and her husband had a very strict timetable for becoming pregnant, so we agreed that if they weren't pregnant after six months we would perform a dye study of the uterus and tubes called a hysterosalpingogram, or HSG (see Figure 2.2). In the meantime her husband went for a semen analysis, which was normal.

Figure 2.2
HYSTEROSALPINGOGRAM (HSG)

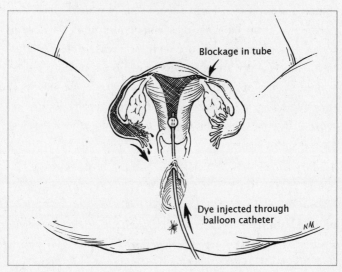

Blockage in tube

Dye injected through balloon catheter

After three more months, I got a call from Priscilla. She had not become pregnant. Priscilla was in her last year of graduate school, and she wanted to complete her pregnancy before graduating and beginning a job. "My schedule is really flexible now and that would make the pregnancy so much easier for me," she said. "I'm worried that I won't have that flexibility when I start a new job."

Once again, we discussed the fact that at least one-third of completely fertile couples are still not pregnant after six months of attempts. But because of their frustration and timetable they wanted to pursue the X-ray dye study (HSG) to assess Priscilla's Fallopian tubes. As it turned out, the HSG revealed that Priscilla had normal female reproductive anatomy. Before we could meet together in my office to discuss the results, Priscilla called me to announce she had become pregnant.

Unless you had a case of pelvic inflammatory disease, often requiring intravenous antibiotics and multiple days of hospitalization, and you have a limited time frame in which you need to become pregnant, I don't suggest you perform an HSG before attempting to conceive on your own for a reasonable period of time. The X-ray dye study is fairly expensive if not covered by your insurance (approximately $500 to $750), can be somewhat uncomfortable, and may lead to surgery to repair tubes or remove scar tissue when you haven't even demonstrated that you have any problem yet.

Other STDs

There are numerous other STDs, such as trichomonas (*Trichomonas vaginalis*), herpes (*herpesvirus*), syphilis (*Treponema pallidum*), and genital warts—also called condyloma acuminatum (human papillomavirus). Although I certainly recommend avoiding these diseases by using condoms (both male and female condoms are now available), they have little, if any, impact on fertility so I won't go into any further detail.

APPENDICITIS

An episode of appendicitis that is treated early in its course will not usually affect fertility. However, a ruptured appendix, when the infected appendix bursts and spills infection into the abdomen and pelvis, can cause damage to the female reproductive organs. If you have had a ruptured appendix, I would recommend the same course of action as for a severe case of PID: try to get pregnant on your own for at least six to nine months before ordering a dye test to assess for possible damage of your tubes. Remember that after one case of PID there is a nearly 90 percent chance that your Fallopian tubes were not significantly damaged, and the chances of damage from a ruptured appendix is probably about the same.

IRREGULAR MENSTRUAL PERIODS

Among the most common reasons that women may have trouble conceiving rapidly are irregular or absent menstrual periods. With irregular cycles, ovulation prediction and accurate timing of intercourse become quite difficult, if not impossible. If your cycles are consistently outside the normal range of 24 to 35 days apart, you should mention this to your physician during your preconceptual counseling visit. Your physician will probably want to do some basic testing to evaluate why your cycles are not regular and whether you're actually ovulating.

The causes of irregular cycles are numerous and could easily fill a chapter or even a book of their own. One cause I will focus on is polycystic ovarian syndrome (PCOS) (formerly referred to as Stein-Leventhal syndrome) because it is the most common identifiable cause of persistently abnormal cycles.

POLYCYSTIC OVARIAN SYNDROME (PCOS)

PCOS is the most common hormonal disorder of reproductive-age women; it affects approximately 5 percent of the population or one in twenty women. Despite this, PCOS remains largely unknown, even by the women who have the syndrome. Fortunately, PCOS has recently received more attention in women's magazines, on talk shows, and in the news media. I guarantee that after reading this section you will be able to identify at least one person you know who has this problem.

PCOS is characterized by:

- irregular menstrual periods;
- unwanted hair growth (examples: facial, chest, around the nipples, below the navel), oily skin, and/or acne;
- being overweight (in more than half of the cases);
- difficulty in becoming pregnant.

The name "polycystic ovaries" is somewhat of a misnomer and a nonspecific term. Women with PCOS have enlarged ovaries with many tiny asymptomatic cysts seen on ultrasound. It also happens that 25 percent of normal women have ovaries that appear polycystic in ultrasound evaluation, so the diagnosis cannot be made by ultrasound appearance alone.

A common misconception is that thin women cannot have PCOS. Although it is true that most women with PCOS are overweight, about one-third of women with PCOS are normal weight for their height. Another misconception is that PCOS can be diagnosed by talking and then doing a physical exam. PCOS is a diagnosis of exclusion, meaning that other diagnoses that could be confused with PCOS need to be ruled out before PCOS is confirmed. Common medical problems that can be confused with PCOS include diabetes and thyroid disease. Less common medical problems that can present in similar ways to PCOS include elevated prolactin, congenital adrenal hyperplasia, and Cushing Syndrome. Your physician must draw blood to make the diagnosis! An ultrasound of the ovaries is also commonly performed.

PCOS Runs in Families

Brenda, 39, came to see me about her problems with obesity, unwanted hair growth, and irregular menstrual periods. Our evaluation revealed that she had PCOS. One of Brenda's major concerns was for her two daughters, ages 10 and 12. Brenda asked me, "What are the chances that they will get PCOS . . . and can PCOS be passed from mother to daughter?" Unfortunately, it does appear that a predisposition for PCOS can be inherited, but the genetic patterns remain unclear. A daughter is estimated to have as high as a 50 percent risk of developing PCOS if her mother was affected.

The exact cause of PCOS has eluded investigators for decades, but recent research indicates that excess insulin production is likely to be a key factor in many women. The majority of overweight women with PCOS seem to have a cellular signaling mechanism for the hormone insulin that does not work efficiently, so that higher levels of insulin are required to achieve a normal response. The excess insulin in PCOS also stimulates the ovaries to produce an overabundance of male-type hormones (for example, testosterone), referred to as androgens. All women produce androgens, but women with PCOS make too much. The excessive androgens and other hormonal irregularities of PCOS lead to the lack of ovulation (resulting in irregular or absent menstrual periods), excessive unwanted hair growth, acne, oily skin, and an increased risk for cardiovascular disease, elevated cholesterol, adult-onset diabetes and diabetes during pregnancy, and cancer of the uterine lining (endometrial cancer). Women with PCOS have diminished fertility mainly because their ovulation is rare and unpredictable.

You have probably heard of the hormone insulin in connection with another disease: diabetes. In fact, the abnormal insulin-signaling mechanism involved in PCOS appears to be similar to the underlying cause of adult-onset diabetes. Many scientists think that PCOS belongs on a spectrum of insulin problems, with PCOS on the mild end and adult-onset diabetes on the severe end. Studies have shown that a large portion of women with PCOS have other family members with adult-onset diabetes mellitus. Women with PCOS need to realize they are predisposed to becoming a diabetic as they age.

Because PCOS affects one in twenty women, it is a very common cause of decreased fertility. In fact, PCOS is the most common hormonal cause of infertility. Women with PCOS often visit their doctors to report irregular bleeding. If a woman with PCOS goes a few months without a menstrual period, her endometrium may build up to a point where irregular bleeding occurs from overgrowth and breakdown of the tissue. This bleeding can be heavy and require hormonal medications or, in severe cases, hospitalization with blood transfusions, or a surgical procedure called dilatation and curettage (D&C). Women with PCOS who have not had a menstrual period for a prolonged period of time will be at greater risk of developing cellular changes in the uterine lining called hyperplasia, which can progress to endometrial cancer if left untreated. When ovulation does occur, the subsequent menstrual flow is often very heavy due to the thickened lining.

Interestingly, it appears that there is a male version of PCOS. Obviously men don't have ovaries, but the genetic problem behind PCOS leads to premature balding in a large percentage of brothers and sons of women affected by PCOS. These men start balding before age 30. The other signs of PCOS, such as unwanted hair growth or acne, are not manifested in men because their bodies naturally produce high levels of male hormones.

Treatment of PCOS

You can see that decreased fertility with PCOS is important, but it's only one of many concerns that need to be addressed. If you suspect you have PCOS, you should consider visiting your obstetrician/gynecologist or a reproductive endocrinologist to be evaluated. Blood tests can help establish the diagnosis, and your doctor can offer you a number of treatment options. However, the diagnosis of PCOS is usually made clinically, through your medical history and a physical exam. Most women will be able to identify themselves as having PCOS merely through the description in this chapter. *In fact, for most women with PCOS, the most effective long-term treatment does not require a doctor's help and can be done at home.*

For most overweight women with PCOS, the most effective treatment and the only true cure is losing weight. A likely theory is that excess weight triggers PCOS by raising insulin levels to a threshold where they stimulate the ovaries to make more male-type hormones, enough to interfere with the normal menstrual cycle. The excess insulin is a powerful hormone, and it encourages the body to preserve its fat stores. This leads to a vicious cycle of insulin-promoting weight gain and excess fat increasing insulin levels. If you have PCOS and have found it extremely difficult to lose weight, you are not alone. If a woman is obese, losing as little as 5 to 10 percent of her body weight can be very effective in breaking the vicious cycle. Many of my overweight PCOS patients have had great success in normalizing their menstrual periods and reversing the other annoying PCOS symptoms after they have lost weight. *Even a modest weight loss of 5 to 10 percent of total body weight has been shown to be enough to allow resumption of normal ovulation and menstrual cycles in many women with PCOS.* Because diabetes and PCOS are similar in their underlying mechanisms of disease, many reproductive endocrinology clinics are encouraging women with PCOS to try a modified diabetic diet to promote a natural reduction in insulin levels. This means decreasing your intake of simple sugars and carbohydrates, while consuming more protein and nonstarchy vegetables.

If you believe you have PCOS and you are overweight, I strongly suggest you read Chapter 6 to plan an effective weight loss and exercise program. Being overweight alone or in combination with PCOS is strongly correlated with reproductive problems, including infertility, miscarriage, and pregnancy complications. Chapter 6 reviews effective weight loss strategies for women with PCOS who want to conceive. There are also a number of best-selling diet books that emphasize an insulin-lowering approach. I will discuss the dietary aspects of PCOS, including some popular diet books, in much greater detail in Chapter 6. I will also review proven, time-tested weight loss strategies for anyone with a weight problem. It is a wonderful idea to visit a Registered Dietician for a consult. However, I suggest you call the office first to make sure the dietician is familiar with PCOS and insulin resistance before making the appointment. If you are in the minority of women with PCOS who are not above the normal weight range for your height, unfortunately weight loss is not the treatment for you.

If you suspect PCOS, especially if you have not had a menstrual period in more than three months or have experienced irregular or excessive menstrual bleeding, you should visit your obstetrician/gynecologist for an evaluation before attempting self-treatment. Metformin (trade name is Glucophage) is an insulin-sensitizing (-lowering) medication first developed for diabetes treatment. Over the last five to ten years it has become popular and widely utilized in women with PCOS to normalize menstrual cycles and facilitate ovulation. Unlike other medications, such as clomiphene citrate or gonadotropins (FSH), metformin does not increase the risk of multiple pregnancy. It appears to work in a more natural way to normalize the balance of hormones and allow cycling to resume in some women. A study by Dr. Stefano Palomba and colleagues, published in the *Journal of Clinical Endocrinology and Metabolism in* 2005, showed that in nonobese women with PCOS, ovulation occurred in two out of three cycles in response to metformin. In obese PCOS women it appears to be a lower rate of response, probably closer to one out of three. In either case, metformin has become a first-line treatment to consider.

PREVIOUS PELVIC SURGERY

Any time you undergo surgery, regardless of the type, scar tissue forms. This is of particular concern with surgery to the female pelvis. Mild scarring in other areas of the body is usually inconsequential, but the ovaries and Fallopian tubes are very delicate organs, and even minimal handling can often leave scar tissue. The scarring can block a Fallopian tube or impede the ovary's ability to release an egg.

The good news is that modern surgical techniques, combined with an awareness of the delicate nature of the female reproductive organs, have minimized the amount of damage done during surgery. Even if you have had an ovary removed in the past due to a cyst or tumor, the remaining ovary and tube should usually be fully functional. *In nearly all cases, no special testing is necessary prior to attempting to conceive on your own.*

HISTORY OF ECTOPIC PREGNANCY

In an ectopic pregnancy, the fertilized egg implants and starts to grow outside the uterus—usually in the Fallopian tube. This is fairly common, affecting 1 to 2 percent of all pregnancies. Ectopic pregnancy is more common in women with damaged Fallopian tubes. The ectopic pregnancy can be a life-threatening emergency if it grows to a size large enough to rupture the Fallopian tube and cause internal bleeding. With modern ultrasound and laboratory technology, and better awareness by emergency room physicians, this condition is diagnosed earlier and treated better.

Until the late 1980s, ectopic pregnancies were always removed surgically. A shift in medical practice occurred around 1990, when it was found that many ectopic pregnancies could be safely treated with a medication called methotrexate, which causes the pregnancy to be absorbed by the body. When surgery is required doctors usually use laparoscopy, a small camera placed into the abdomen, to perform more conservative, outpatient surgery.

In the past, ectopic pregnancy usually resulted in the loss of the Fallopian tube on the affected side. This reduced the fertility of the woman, but if the other tube was functional, she didn't usually become infertile. With modern surgical techniques it is often the case that at the time of surgery to remove the ectopic pregnancy a tube may be able to be saved rather than removed. In the last decade, conservative surgery or treatment with methotrexate has enabled more women to preserve both their

Fallopian tubes. The likelihood of permanent infertility after a single ectopic pregnancy is now extremely low, unless it was due to previous damage by a process that affected both your Fallopian tubes (such as PID, endometriosis, or an extensive surgical procedure).

After one of my patients used methotrexate to successfully treat her ectopic pregnancy she asked me, "How do I know an ectopic pregnancy won't happen next time too?" Keep in mind that after one episode of ectopic pregnancy, you are at higher risk to have another one in the future. However, the odds of a normal pregnancy are still greatly in your favor. Studies have shown that, with contemporary treatments for ectopic pregnancy, about 80 percent of postectopic Fallopian tubes are not blocked by scar tissue caused from either the pregnancy or its treatment.

It is appropriate to be optimistic that you will have a successful pregnancy next time. Unless you have had a previous medical problem that predisposes both your tubes to being damaged, or damage to the other tube is noted at the time of surgery, *you shouldn't have to evaluate your tubal function prior to attempting to conceive again on your own.* My only recommendation is that you perform home pregnancy tests to make sure you discover your pregnancy early on. Notify your obstetrician of your history of ectopic pregnancy. Your doctor will probably want you to come in for blood testing initially and then an early ultrasound—by about six weeks after your last menstrual period—to make sure the pregnancy is in the correct place.

OVARIAN CYSTS

In Chapter 1, I discussed how a woman generates a follicle, a fluid-filled sac or cyst, on the ovary that contains the egg to be released that month. Ovulation occurs when special enzymes create a hole in the wall of the follicle, allowing the fluid inside to flow out and bring the egg with it. After ovulation, the collapsed follicle re-forms into a fluid-filled sac called the corpus luteum cyst. This corpus luteum cyst persists during the next two weeks or so after ovulation in all women.

The reason I have just reviewed this is to emphasize that women normally make two different cysts each month, one called a follicle and the other called the corpus luteum. When women say they have had cysts in the past, they are describing cysts as some unusual occurrence. Most often those cysts are merely persistent follicles or a corpus luteum and are benign, although they can sometimes rupture (or grow to abnormal size), causing pain. In women of reproductive age, however, it is uncommon to find a cyst that is not benign and that will not disappear on its own within six to eight weeks.

Unless the cysts have required surgery or were not benign, you can be almost certain that a past history of forming cysts will have no impact on your fertility. Even with surgery, most women will have preserved fertility postoperatively. Don't confuse ovarian cysts with polycystic ovarian syndrome (PCOS); they are two completely separate issues.

HISTORY OF ELECTIVE ABORTION

Americans have more abortions than any other industrialized nation in the world. Between 1.5 and 2 million women undergo elective termination of pregnancies each year in the United States. This means that a large proportion of women will have had a history of at least one elective abortion prior to starting their families.

Occasionally I get questions about the relationship between an elective abortion and fertility. In general, the answer is that there is very little risk of damaging the female reproductive organs during the procedure. An abortion is usually performed using an outpatient surgical technique called a dilatation and evacuation. As long as there were no complications, such as an infection, cervical tearing, or uterine perforation, I wouldn't worry. Scarring of the uterine cavity can occasionally occur after the procedure, but this would usually cause the woman's menstrual period to become significantly lighter or disappear. *Following an abortion, if the procedure was uncomplicated and your menstrual bleeding was similar to prior menstrual periods, then you have no reason for concern.* A history of abortion reveals one reassuring piece of information about a woman's body: she has proven her ability to become pregnant.

Recently a variety of nonsurgical methods, including oral medications and vaginal suppositories, have become available for terminating pregnancy. Two of the new drugs are misoprostol (Cytotec) and RU-486 (Mifepristone). They are not in widespread use right now, but are likely to be in the near future. I am unaware of any studies that compare the risks of infertility from an abortion induced by either of these medications to the surgical techniques. It seems logical to conclude that substituting a medication for a surgical procedure would be even less likely to damage the female reproductive organs and have any impact on future fertility.

PREVIOUS MISCARRIAGE

Miscarriage is an intensely personal event. Some couples choose not to share their sadness and disappointment with anyone, but often a couple will seek support from family members or a close friend. Because couples share their history of a miscarriage with few people, it seems to be a relatively uncommon occurrence. In fact, if home pregnancy tests are used very early, an estimated 20 percent of all pregnancies will be shown to end in miscarriage. If sensitive blood tests for pregnancy are used shortly after implantation of the embryo, then some studies have indicated that one-third or more of pregnancies do not progress. This means that miscarriage is in fact extremely common, and women using reliable mass-marketed pregnancy test kits are more likely to realize when an early miscarriage has taken place.

Because the occurrence of a single early miscarriage is so common, you need to realize that it may occur again. After one miscarriage the risk of another miscarriage is not significantly higher, so the odds are still greatly in your favor that all will go well. Keep in mind that even if you have had two miscarriages—and no prior live-born baby—the chance that you will have a normal, healthy pregnancy with the next attempt is about 60 percent. If you've ever had a normal pregnancy in the past, then your chances of delivering a healthy baby after having two miscarriages is about 75 percent. If you have only had one previous miscarriage, it is appropriate to be very optimistic that the next pregnancy will be normal. If you have had two miscarriages, I think it would be prudent to see

Paula and her husband, Steve, came to see me for a follow-up appointment a few weeks after they had a miscarriage. "I don't think I could go through that again," Paula said with great sadness in her voice. "I've never been so disappointed in my life. What can we do to try to make sure it doesn't happen again?"

your obstetrician/gynecologist or a reproductive endocrinologist for an evaluation.

My wife, Kara, had an early miscarriage with our first pregnancy. After our miscarriage, Kara and I racked our brains trying to think about what we could have done to cause the miscarriage. This is exactly what I tell all my patients *not* to do.

The most common cause of miscarriage is a random genetic abnormality. At least 50 percent of early miscarriages are believed to be due to chromosomal abnormalities. This is just plain bad luck in most cases. My only recommendation is this: if you have had a single early miscarriage, make sure to read Chapter 3, "Preconceptional Care." There are some things a couple can do to reduce the chance of miscarriage, including treating certain infections, quitting cigarettes, optimizing medical conditions, avoiding exposure to certain environmental toxins, and eating a healthy diet. Otherwise there is really nothing to be done about the genetic mistakes that cause most miscarriages.

Depending on your age you might also want to read Chapter 10, which describes the correlation between age and the rate of chromosomal abnormalities and miscarriage. Not that any of us can do anything about our age, but it emphasizes a realistic understanding and expectation for pregnancies at all ages. As I mentioned above, there are things that can be done at any age to minimize your risk for miscarriage, and these recommendations are reviewed in Chapter 10.

CONCLUSIONS

You have probably been affected by one or more of the topics discussed in this chapter. The truth is that most fertile women will be affected by at least one of the common female gynecological problems that can affect fertility, but the vast majority of couples will never have any significant fertility problem from any of these issues. Although it is easy to become concerned, I hope this review was educational and has left you with a feeling of optimism. In those cases that can have long-term effects on fertility, such as polycystic ovarian syndrome and endometriosis, you do have options and treatments available to maximize your fertility, and you should discuss these with your physician. As you read further in the book many of these issues will be reviewed again in more detail and more specific strategies will be offered.

3

Preconceptional Care

CREATING A HEALTHY BABY

THE one thing all couples reading this book want most is to have a healthy baby. The vast majority of couples will have a healthy baby regardless of whether they have preconceptional care, but some of the birth defects that do occur are preventable. Awareness of the importance of preconceptional counseling and making the appropriate interventions will increase the chances of having a healthy baby.

A baby begins to form organs about 17 days after fertilization, which is only a few days after a woman would be able to discover she is pregnant. So, by the time you visit your doctor for your first prenatal visit, many of your baby's organ systems will have already been formed, and it will be too late to intervene with many important preventative measures. If you make sure you receive proper nutrition and immunization against certain diseases, avoid harmful medications, deal effectively with your preexisting medical conditions, receive appropriate genetic counseling, and avoid certain environmental exposures *before you become pregnant*, you can help reduce your baby's chances for birth defects to the lowest possible level. According to the American College of Obstetricians and Gynecologists, nearly one in twenty babies (4.5 percent) has a birth defect recognized by age five. A significant proportion of these fetal malformations, and many maternal complications, can be prevented by appropriate preconceptional care. Contrary to the popular saying, what you don't know can hurt you and your baby when it comes to preconceptional care.

The idea of preconceptional care hasn't been around that long, and recommendations are changing rapidly as experts focus more attention on this vital subject. *In a perfect world all couples would go to their physician for a preconceptional visit before they start trying to get pregnant.* Some physicians are not as up-to-date on preconceptional recommendations as others, so couples must also be educated to make sure they're not missing any of the latest information or recommendations.

Most of the recommendations in this chapter regarding nutrition, immunization, medications, and environmental exposures are directed to the female partner. *This does not mean, however, that only the woman should go in for the preconceptional visit.* The pregnancy will deeply affect both partners, and both of you should know about the changes that should take place in your medical treatment and lifestyle. There are many things men can do to improve their fertility and the health of their babies, and this information is reviewed in Chapter 8. Additionally, most of the important considerations—such as lifestyle changes or professional and financial implications—involve both future parents and will require a reasonable level of agreement *before you become pregnant.*

NUTRITION AND BIRTH DEFECTS

Folic Acid

One of the easiest and most effective things a woman can do preconceptionally to ensure the health of her baby is to take folic acid (folate) supplements. By taking one multivitamin with 400 micrograms (0.4 milligrams) of folic acid a day, starting before conception, a woman can reduce the chance that her baby will suffer a neural tube defect by at least 50 percent. Other less-well-known benefits of folic acid include a significant reduction in fetal urinary tract and cardiovascular defects, limb deficiencies, and gastrointestinal malformations.

Spinal cord and brain malformations, called neural tube defects, are common, afflicting between one and two of every 1,000 live births in the United States. Worldwide there are about a half-million cases of neural tube defects, with 4,000 of these occurring in the U.S. This category includes such birth defects as spina bifida, encephalocele, and anencephaly. *The brain and spinal cord have undergone significant development by the time a woman is six weeks pregnant* (six weeks from the last menstrual period), *so the best advice is to begin your prenatal vitamins before you become pregnant.*

In 1992 the Public Health Service issued a recommendation that all women of childbearing age who may become pregnant consume 400 micrograms of folic acid per day. A survey conducted in 1997 by the March of Dimes evaluated the knowledge of folic acid and birth defects among women of childbearing age in the United States. Sixty-six percent of women said they had heard of folic acid, but of these women only 16 percent reported that they knew folic acid prevented birth defects and only 9 percent understood that folic acid had to be started *before* the pregnancy. This survey shows how long it may take to disseminate important public health information to the population.

Women with no risk factors for neural tube defects should consume 400 to 600 micrograms (0.4 to 0.6 milligrams) of folic acid per day beginning prior to conception. Look at the label on your vitamin bottle and make sure there is enough folic acid in your daily dosage. If there isn't enough, don't take extra vitamins to make up the difference. As you will see below, too much of some of the other vitamins found in the tablets can be harmful.

Recent studies have shown that as many as one in seven families carries a genetic mutation that makes them deficient in their ability to absorb or use the folic acid in their diet. If you or your partner has a parent or sibling with a neural tube defect or if one of your siblings has a child with a neural tube defect, this may indicate that your family is at higher risk. Siblings of women who had a baby with a neural tube defect have about a 5 percent incidence of having a baby with a neural tube defect. You should consult your doctor for advice about how much folic acid you should be taking preconceptionally if you believe that your family might be at higher risk for neural tube defects. *If you have had a previously affected child then you should take 4 milligrams of folic acid per day beginning one month prior to conception.* This is ten times the normal dose recommended. If you are in the high-risk category, you will need a supplement for folic acid alone so that you don't exceed recommended daily doses of other vitamins found in multivitamins. Ten prenatal multivitamins would be required to make up the 4-milligram dose, but excessive multivitamin intake puts the baby at risk for birth defects from high levels of vitamins (such as vitamin A); therefore, the 4-milligram dose should be taken as a separate supplement apart from the prenatal multivitamin. However, women should not take more than 1 milligram of folic acid each day without their doctor's advice.

Oral contraceptives can decrease the amount of folic acid in your system despite appropriate levels of supplementation. I recommend that if you are taking oral contraceptives up until the time you are going to try to get pregnant, you should take 1 milligram of folic acid per day, rather than the 0.4 milligrams normally recommended. Many people want to supplement their nutrition "naturally," rather than take a pill each day. If you want to try to add folic acid to your diet, you have many options. Folic acid is found in leafy green vegetables, asparagus, broccoli, beans, lentils, dried peas, organ meats, orange juice, and fortified breakfast cereals. However, it's difficult to get the recommended daily allowance of folic acid through diet alone. Dietary sources of folic acid are not as bioavailable, meaning that even if a helping of food contains a certain amount of folic acid, the body isn't able to use it all. In fact, you must consume twice as much dietary folic acid to equal the folic acid found in a vitamin pill or supplemented breakfast cereal. *This means that it takes food containing 800 micrograms (0.8 milligrams) of folic acid for the body to remove the 400 micrograms (0.4 milligrams) required each day.*

All of the research studies have used folic acid in a pill form to prevent neural tube defects. One can assume folic acid from natural sources would be equally efficacious, but no studies have been performed to confirm this. Additionally, it is difficult to assess the exact amount of folic acid taken in by the diet. For these reasons, the Centers for Disease Control (CDC), the Institute of Medicine, and the U.S. Public Health Service recommend a synthetic source (vitamin supplement) for folic acid rather than a dietary source.

Analogous to the fortification of vitamin D in milk or the addition of fluoride to water, beginning in January 1998 all breads, pastas, rice, and other grain products were required to be fortified with folic acid. Now each 100 milligrams of grain must have 0.14 milligrams of folic acid. This will increase the average American woman's folic acid intake by 100 micrograms (0.1 milligrams) per day. With these new rules, the U.S. Food and Drug Administration hopes to improve dietary intake of folic acid in the future.

Vitamin A

The deregulation of nutritional supplements created a multibillion-dollar industry, and the popularity of vitamin and mineral supplementation soared. It seems like everyone is taking a supplement of some sort, and frequently "megadosing." But many people don't realize that you can get too much of a good thing, and this is especially true when it comes to preconceptional and early pregnancy nutrition.

Vitamin A is a popular supplement for general health. Many Americans "megadose" on pills containing vitamin A. This nutrient has become a popular supplement for promotion of skin health and is contained in many skin creams and lotions. Retin-A, a topical medication, and Accutane, a pill (also known by their generic names as isotretinoin, tretinoin, retinoic acid, or vitamin A acid), are popular prescription medications, similar in structure to vitamin A, that many people use for severe acne.

The recommended daily allowance for vitamin A is 5,000 IU (or 800 µg retinol equivalents). Recent studies have shown that *dosages in the range of 10,000 to 25,000 IU can cause birth defects*. The exact threshold IU level for concern has not been clearly established, so *pregnant women and women trying to get pregnant should not exceed the recommended daily allowance, or 5,000 IU, for vitamin A.* Check your multivitamin bottle to see how much vitamin A is included, and also look at other products you are using, especially skin products, to see if you may be getting other sources of vitamin A. Skin can absorb significant levels of vitamin A into the bloodstream. I recommend discontinuing these products prior to attempting to become pregnant.

The good news is that beta-carotene, the precursor to vitamin A found in vegetables and fruits, does not appear to cause vitamin A toxicity. So you shouldn't be able to overdose on the vitamin A in fruits and vegetables. People who eat a lot of animal liver consume excessive amounts of vitamin A, but it is not certain whether this is associated with an increased risk for birth defects.

Zinc

Zinc deficiency has been linked to a higher incidence of birth defects. Strenuous exercisers may be zinc deficient because zinc leaves the body through the sweat, so these individuals should be careful to adequately supplement their zinc. Oral contraceptive use also can decrease levels of zinc, so if you plan on using birth-control pills up until the month you are going to try to get pregnant, then make sure that you are eating a well-balanced diet and supplementing your zinc with a prenatal vitamin. Vegetarians may also have difficulty obtaining enough zinc without taking a prenatal vitamin because very little zinc is found in plant sources. The dietary fertility challenges for vegetarians are discussed in detail in Chapter 7.

Zinc lozenges have grown very popular these days to protect against "catching a cold." But excessive zinc decreases copper intake and may lead to copper deficiency, which can result in complications during pregnancy. I recommend supplementing a healthy diet with a daily prenatal multivitamin to ensure adequate levels of zinc, but avoiding the lozenges.

Other Vitamins/Minerals

Vitamins D, E, and C have also been implicated in birth defects if either inadequate or excessive levels are present in the mother. As we learn more about the role of nutrition and birth defects, recommendations will certainly be altered. My advice to you would be that until more is known about this subject, take one multivitamin with 400 to 600 micrograms of folic acid daily and make sure the levels of other vitamins and minerals meet but do not exceed the recommended dietary allowances (see Figures 3.1 A and B). The key is having the right amount—not too much or too little—of the essential vitamins and minerals. Vitamins marketed as "prenatal" in pharmacies and grocery stores should have exactly the levels you are looking for. Further supplementation is unnecessary and can be dangerous. Beyond that, just consume a healthy diet, and you should be doing everything necessary. In general, it's very hard to consume toxic levels of vitamins and minerals through your diet alone. Usually the concern is either inadequate levels of vitamins and minerals, or excessive vitamin and mineral supplementation through megadosing.

The relationship between nutrition and birth defects should be clear at this point. The role of nutrition in how quickly a woman will become pregnant will be reviewed in Chapter 7, and the important dietary considerations for optimal male fertility will be reviewed in Chapter 8.

Figure 3.1A
DIETARY REFERENCE INTAKES TO APPLY PRECONCEPTIONALLY

Life-Stage Group	Calcium (mg/d)	Phosphorus (mg/d)	Magnesium (mg/d)	Vitamin D (μg/d)[a,b]	Fluoride (mg/d)	Thiamin (mg/d)	Riboflavin (mg/d)	Niacin (mg/d)[c]	Vitamin B₆ (mg/d)	Folate (μg/d)[d]	Vitamin B₁₂ (μg/d)	Pantothenic Acid (mg/d)	Biotin (μg/d)	Choline[e] (mg/d)
Pregnancy														
≤18 yr	1,300*	1,250*	400	5*	3*	1.4	1.4	18	1.9	600[g,h]	2.6	6*	30*	450*
19–30 yr	1,000*	700	350	5*	3*	1.4	1.4	18	1.9	600[g,h]	2.6	6*	30*	450*
31–50 yr	1,000*	700	360	5*	3*	1.4	1.4	18	1.9	600[g,h]	2.6	6*	30*	450*

NOTE: This table presents Recommended Dietary Allowances (RDAs) in **bold type** and Adequate Intakes (AIs) in ordinary type followed by an asterisk (*). RDAs and AIs may both be used as goals for individual intake. RDAs are set to meet the needs of almost all (97 to 98 percent) individuals in a group. For healthy breastfed infants, the AI is the mean intake. The AI for other life-stage and gender groups is believed to cover needs of all individuals in the group, but lack of data or uncertainty in the data prevent being able to specify with confidence the percentage of individuals covered by this intake.

[a] As cholecalciferol. 1 μg cholecalciferol = 40 IU vitamin D.

[b] In the absence of adequate exposure to sunlight.

[c] As niacin equivalents (NE). 1 mg of niacin = 60 mg of tryptophan; 0–6 months = preformed niacin (not NE).

[d] As dietary folate equivalents (DFE). 1 DFE = 1 μg food folate = 0.6 μg of folic acid from fortified food or as a supplement consumed with food = 0.5 μg of a supplement taken on an empty stomach.

[e] Although AIs have been set for choline, there are few data to assess whether a dietary supply of choline is needed at all stages of the life cycle, and it may be that the choline requirement can be met by endogenous synthesis at some of these stages.

[g] In view of evidence linking folate intake with neural tube defects in the fetus, it is recommended that all women capable of becoming pregnant consume 400 μg from supplements or fortified foods in addition to intake of food folate from a varied diet.

[h] It is assumed that women will continue consuming 400 μg from supplements or fortified food until their pregnancy is confirmed and they enter prenatal care, which ordinarily occurs after the end of the periconceptional period—the critical time for formation of the neural tube.

Figure 3.1B

RECOMMENDED DIETARY ALLOWANCES TO APPLY PRECONCEPTIONALLY

FOOD AND NUTRITION BOARD, NATIONAL ACADEMY OF SCIENCES–NATIONAL RESEARCH COUNCIL
RECOMMENDED DIETARY ALLOWANCES,[a] Revised 1989 (Abridged)

Designed for the maintenance of good nutrition of practically all healthy people in the United States

Category	Protein (g)	Vitamin A (μg RE)[b]	Vitamin E (mg α-TE)[d]	Vitamin K (μg)	Vitamin C (mg)	Iron (mg)	Zinc (mg)	Iodine (μg)	Selenium (μg)
Pregnant	60	800	10	65	70	30	15	175	65

NOTE: This table does not include nutrients for which Dietary Reference Intakes have recently been established (see *Dietary Reference Intakes for Calcium, Phosphorus, Magnesium, Vitamin D, and Fluoride* [1997] and *Dietary Reference Intakes for Thiamin, Riboflavin, Niacin, Vitamin B₆, Folate, Vitamin B₁₂, Pantothenic Acid, Biotin, and Choline* [1998]).

[a] The allowances, expressed as average daily intakes over time, are intended to provide for individual variations among most normal persons as they live in the United States under usual environmental stresses. Diets should be based on a variety of common foods in order to provide other nutrients for which human requirements have been less well defined.

[c] Retinol equivalents. 1 retinol equivalent = 1 μg retinol or 6 μg β-carotene.

[d] α-Tocopherol equivalents. 1 mg d-α tocopherol = 1 α-TE.

IMMUNIZATIONS/INFECTIOUS DISEASES

Rubella

One of the first major breakthroughs in preconceptional care occurred in 1969 with the release of a rubella vaccine. Rubella infection during pregnancy can result in congenital rubella syndrome in the fetus, which can cause serious malformations. Nearly all U.S. children receive vaccinations for rubella, but immunity to rubella can be lost over time. For this reason all women are routinely tested for immunity to rubella every time they become pregnant. However, if a woman is found to be nonimmune, she will remain at risk for getting rubella throughout the pregnancy because it isn't considered safe to give the vaccine during pregnancy.

You should be tested for rubella before pregnancy so that if you're not immune to the virus, you can be safely vaccinated before becoming pregnant. Many doctors are accustomed to testing women after they have become pregnant, because it used to be rare for a woman to see her physician in preparation for becoming pregnant. There's a good chance you will need to ask your doctor to test for rubella immunity when you visit him or her at your preconceptional counseling visit. In fact, my sister-in-law's physician told her it would be fine to have her rubella immunity checked after she got pregnant, not understanding that she could avoid a possible case of congenital rubella syndrome by simply performing the test prior to the pregnancy and immunizing if necessary.

The Centers for Disease Control (CDC) recommends that women of childbearing age continue to use a reliable form of birth control for three months after receiving a rubella vaccination. The CDC has collected data on 307 infants born to mothers who received the rubella vaccine for up to three months before conception or during the first trimester. There were no defects consistent with a rubella infection noted in the babies. It seems that the risk of a fetal malformation from getting pregnant soon after a rubella vaccination is extremely low. Nevertheless, optimally, you should plan ahead so that you can receive a rubella vaccine three months before attempting to become pregnant.

Chicken Pox

Are you sure you had the chicken pox as a child? If you're not sure, call your mother or father and ask them if they remember. Even if you do not remember having the infection the vast majority of you will have had it. If there is any question, then ask your doctor to draw blood for a varicella titer. *Varicella* is the medical term for the chicken pox. A varicella titer will indicate whether or not you had the infection and continue to have immunity. The varicella virus can cause congenital varicella syndrome in the baby, which is a constellation of congenital malformations consisting of limb and eye deformities and mental retardation.

If you find you never had chicken pox, you can now receive a vaccine for varicella. *I would recommend this vaccine for any woman considering pregnancy who didn't get chicken pox as a child*. As with the rubella vaccine, you should wait for three months after receiving the immunization before trying to become pregnant.

Hepatitis

At the time of delivery a baby can acquire the Hepatitis B infection from an infected mother. A significant percentage of

Figure 3.2

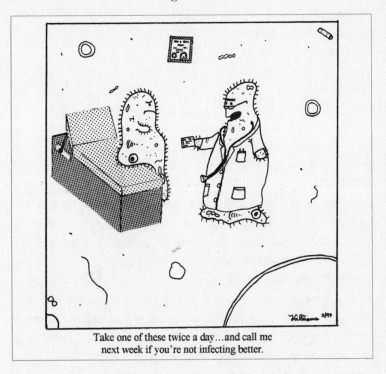

Take one of these twice a day...and call me
next week if you're not infecting better.

these babies will become chronically infected, and the infection can ultimately be fatal. Hepatitis B is most commonly found in health-care workers and among people who engage in high-risk sexual and social behaviors. Most health-care workers are offered the Hepatitis B vaccination; any health-care workers considering pregnancy should get it. Those individuals who participate in high-risk sexual behaviors or intravenous drug use should also consider the Hepatitis B vaccination.

Hepatitis C can also be transmitted to the baby during labor; however, there is currently no vaccine available for Hepatitis C.

Hepatitis C causes similar effects to infected babies as Hepatitis B, but progression of the disease to liver failure and hepatic cancer is more common with Hepatitis C.

HIV

HIV testing is now offered to all pregnant women. Since you will have an HIV test performed once you are pregnant, you might as well have it done *before* you get pregnant. HIV is so common these days that it is naive for people to think it can't possibly happen to them. I've had too many heartbreaking conversations with women who have had no risk factors and who were "mutually monogamous" with their partner.

Would it change your decision about having a baby if you knew you were HIV positive? Even if you answered no to that question, you should still get an HIV test once you're pregnant. There are many excellent drugs that can be used to suppress the HIV virus during pregnancy, drastically reducing your chance of transmitting the infection to your baby. It is nothing less than irresponsible to refuse an HIV test at the beginning of the pregnancy. If the HIV is left untreated during the pregnancy, you are substantially increasing the chances your baby will become HIV positive.

Syphilis

Syphilis is a sexually transmitted disease that is often asymptomatic and can be present in your body for many years. Syphilis can infect the fetus, causing fetal malformations and even death. All women are screened for syphilis once they are pregnant, but whether you suspect the infection or not I would recommend testing prior to pregnancy so that the disease can be treated before you get pregnant.

Gonorrhea/Chlamydia

These sexually transmitted diseases can be responsible for early pregnancy loss and decreased fertility. If you suspect you may have acquired a sexually transmitted disease, see your doctor or local clinic or health department for testing. Common symptoms for both gonorrhea and chlamydia include increased vaginal discharge (especially yellow or greenish in color), lower abdominal/pelvic pain, and pain or burning with urination. The most common initial symptom is a heavier discharge, which is usually followed later by lower abdominal/pelvic pain and fever and/or chills. As with syphilis, testing for gonorrhea and chlamydia is commonly done on all women once they are pregnant. Once again, I recommend you have these tests done at your preconceptional visit to your doctor so that treatment can be completed before you get pregnant.

Tuberculosis

Once a common bacterial infection in the United States, tuberculosis infections became much less common after the introduction of antibiotics. Recently, tuberculosis has made a dramatic resurgence. Health-care workers, people who have been in contact with infected individuals, foreign travelers and immigrants, alcoholics, the elderly, people from lower socioeconomic levels, drug abusers, and HIV-positive individuals are all at higher risk for getting tuberculosis.

Tuberculosis is another infection that is tested for in many pregnant women. An active tuberculosis infection is usually fairly obvious, with chronic coughing, fever and chills, night sweats, and malaise. However, tuberculosis can be carried in your body for many years without any symptoms. *Once again, if you go see your physician preconceptionally, ask if you are in a high-risk group for tuberculosis, and if you are, then request a tuberculosis skin test.* If you have a positive test you will need a chest X-ray and likely will have to take medications for at least six months. If you turn out to have tuberculosis, it would certainly be better to have the X-ray and complete all the medications before becoming pregnant.

Toxoplasmosis

Toxoplasmosis is a parasitic infection that can be transmitted from mother to fetus, resulting in serious birth defects. Humans usually acquire the parasite through the consumption of infected raw or undercooked meat or from contact with cat feces, while cats become infected with toxoplasmosis by hunting mice. Cats and humans can be infected and not show any significant signs or symptoms.

If you have an indoor cat, the chance of your cat acquiring toxoplasmosis is insignificant, unless there are mice in your house. But if your cat has been in contact with mice at any time in the past, it could have become infected at that time and can transmit the disease later. *Women trying to get pregnant and pregnant women should avoid cleaning a cat's litter box.*

Cat owners and people who handle raw meat or consume undercooked meat are at highest risk for being infected with toxoplasmosis. If you are in one of these groups, you should discuss testing with your physician at the preconceptional visit.

Cytomegalovirus (CMV)

Cytomegalovirus is a common infection, and nearly half of adults have had this viral infection in the past. CMV during pregnancy can result in damage to the fetal brain and liver, among other problems. You may be asking yourself, "If CMV is so common, then why haven't I heard about it before?" The reason is that, outside of pregnancy and childhood, the CMV infection does not usually cause any problems worse than the symptoms of a common cold. In fact, one of those times you called in sick to work because you had a cold or flu could have been CMV.

If you work in child care or health care, especially with pediatrics or dialysis units, mention this to your physician at your preconceptional counseling visit. There is testing available to see if you have been infected with CMV in the past. If you had CMV before, you cannot become infected again. If you test negative for previous CMV exposure, you and your doctor can discuss strategies to avoid this infection during pregnancy. Unfortunately there is no vaccine available for CMV. Frequent hand washing and avoiding high-risk groups, such as groups of children, are all that is available at the present time.

Bacterial Vaginosis

In Chapter 1, I emphasized the importance of maintaining the normal balance of vaginal bacteria. In Chapter 2, I reviewed the most recent information regarding the effects of a vaginal infection called bacterial vaginosis on fertility, ectopic pregnancy, and miscarriage. To refresh your memory, bacterial vaginosis results from the overgrowth of certain types of bacteria in the vagina, causing inflammation of the vagina, a "fishy" odor, a thin, milky discharge, vaginal pH changes, and, less commonly, vaginal irritation. This infection is not considered a sexually transmitted disease and is acquired in a similar manner to a yeast infection.

The medical community now recognizes the important relationship between bacterial vaginosis and miscarriage and preterm labor. At the present time, there are no studies that examine the relationship between bacterial vaginosis, or other causes of prolonged changes in the vaginal pH, and delayed conception. It seems quite plausible that processes that change the vaginal pH and cause low-grade inflammation could result in a hostile environment for the sperm, decreasing fertility, in addition to miscarriage and preterm labor risks.

Unlike a yeast infection, which you can treat yourself with an over-the-counter antifungal cream, bacterial vaginosis requires a prescription antibiotic. You should contact your doctor if you suspect bacterial vaginosis, in order to be treated before you become pregnant. Because the infection is frequently asymptomatic, I suggest all women have a preconceptional screening test for bacterial vaginosis.

Figure 3.3

Laboratory Tests to Order Before Pregnancy to Evaluate for Past or Present Infections

- **Rubella titer**—Immunization is available.
- **Varicella titer (chicken pox)**—Immunization is available.
- **HIV**—Treatment is available to minimize the chances that the baby will be infected.
- **Syphilis**—Treatment is available to eliminate the infection.
- **Hepatitis B and C**—Immunization for Hepatitis B is available.
- **Tuberculosis**—Immunization is produced but not used in the United States. Effective antibiotics are available in most cases.
- **Gonorrhea and chlamydia**—Treatment is available to eliminate the infection.

- **Toxoplasmosis**—Treatment is available to eliminate the infection.
- **Cytomegalovirus (CMV)**—No treatment is available; avoiding infection is the only option.
- **Bacterial vaginosis**—Treatment is available to eliminate the infection.

MEDICAL PROBLEMS

There are a number of medical conditions a mother may have that can lead to congenital malformations in the child. The best example of this is the mother with poorly controlled diabetes, who has a two to three times greater risk of having a baby with a birth defect. As in the case of folic acid deficiency, by the time a diabetic mother goes to her physician's office for her first prenatal visit, birth defects may have already occurred. The offspring of mothers with poorly controlled diabetes have higher risks of heart malformations, spinal and limb defects, and other problems. By gaining tight control of the blood sugars *prior to pregnancy* and closely monitoring blood sugar levels, especially during the first trimester, diabetics lower the risk of birth defects to nearly the same as that of nondiabetic mothers. There are some maternal medical conditions that may worsen with pregnancy, leading to potential risks for both the mother and her baby. Significant heart valve disease, primary pulmonary hypertension, and congestive heart failure are some examples. Like diabetes, other medical disorders can cause problems for the fetus if they are not properly monitored and controlled. Seizure disorders that are not adequately controlled may have adverse effects on the fetus. Additionally, many chronic medical conditions in the mother do not affect the baby per se, but the medications used to treat the disorder can cause congenital anomalies.

If you have any chronic medical disorder, especially if you are on any medications, consult your physician before becoming pregnant to discuss a plan to maximize your health and minimize adverse fetal effects.

MEDICATIONS

If you or your partner are taking any medications daily, especially if prescribed, talk to your doctor about whether it is safe to attempt to get pregnant while taking the drug. It is also a good idea to ask your physician about any medications you may take sporadically, such as over-the-counter, or nonprescription, treatments for pain, allergies, stomach upset, cold and flu, or other popular medications. Many nonprescription drugs may have adverse effects on conception or early pregnancy, so don't assume that because a medication is sold without a prescription it is safe to take at the time of conception. A good example of a prescription medication to be avoided is Accutane (also known as isotretinoin), which is used to treat severe acne and causes severe fetal abnormalities. It's best to wait at least one month after your last usage before trying to conceive. Call your doctor's office to ask about the safety of any medication you might be taking, whether it is prescription or nonprescription. Also see Figure 3.6 later in this chapter for information on easy access to databases on chemical and drug exposures during early pregnancy.

GENETIC COUNSELING

Since the discovery of the structure of DNA in the 1950s, research into genetics has grown at an amazing rate. The

Figure 3.4
CHROMOSOMES, GENES, AND DNA

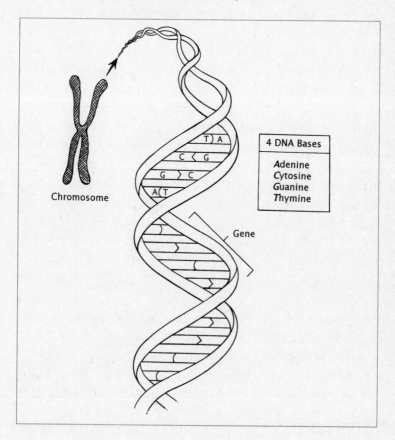

Chromosome

4 DNA Bases

Adenine
Cytosine
Guanine
Thymine

Gene

Human Genome Project is a massive effort to sequence all the genes present in our chromosomes, so we will eventually have the codes for all the processes that occur in our bodies. With this research have come many insights into common genetic diseases. In some cases tests can now be offered preconceptionally for specific genetic diseases. More amazing is that some genetic diseases can now be cured using various forms of gene therapy, and the number of treatable genetic diseases keeps growing. In fact, the future of medical therapy will be at the genetic level, preventing diseases before they occur.

Genetic counseling may be applied preconceptionally, during the pregnancy, or after delivery. Genetic counseling refers to the assessment of the risk of conceiving a child with a genetic disease and discussions of testing and treatment available. Based on your personal and family history, risks can be assigned to the possibility of your offspring being affected by a genetic problem. Genetic diseases may be inherited from a parent or arise at random from new mutations in a child's genes.

Figure 3.5
RISK FACTORS FOR GENETIC DISORDERS

- Mother will be 35 years of age or older at the time the baby will be born
- Family history of birth defects (either partner)
- Family history of diseases that seem to "run in the family"
- Personal history of a previous child affected with a birth defect or inherited disease
- History of a child in the family that died unexpectedly
- Two or more previous miscarriages
- A family member who is "slow" or "learning disabled"
- Personal history of a disease that could be inherited by your offspring
- Ethnic background: African-American, Jewish (especially Eastern European), Mediterranean, French Canadian, or Southeast Asian

Inherited Disorders

Some disorders can be inherited, meaning the disease is passed down in the genes from parent to child. Common examples include sickle cell disease, cystic fibrosis, some forms of mental retardation, and muscular dystrophy. When a disease "runs" in a family, some family members will be afflicted, whereas others will have no symptoms but may or may not be carriers of the disease, meaning they can pass it on to their children. Frequently couples do not realize that a specific disorder present in their family is a genetic disease and can be passed to their offspring.

If you think there's a chance that your family might carry a serious inherited disorder, or if you meet any of the risk factors for genetic disorders in Figure 3.5, I recommend that you meet with your doctor or a genetic counselor before your pregnancy to uncover a possible pattern of disease inheritance. Testing can give a couple information to help them in their decision making. Some diseases can only be carried by one sex, and reasonably good technology is now available for sorting sperm to allow a couple a very high probability of having a child with the desired sex (see Chapter 11).

More commonly, couples can use the information they've learned to discuss what may occur. It's better to have some idea of the possibilities and options beforehand, than to be shocked to find out your newborn is affected by an inherited disease. In some instances, I have had patients who decided to adopt or use donor sperm or eggs due to the seriousness of the possible disorder. The latest technology, called preimplantation genetic diagnosis, uses a modification of in vitro fertilization to allow couples to select only healthy embryos for their pregnancy. This virtually guarantees a healthy baby.

Random Chromosomal Disorders

Other genetic disorders are not inherited but occur randomly. When the sperm and egg meet, they each contribute approximately half of the DNA that makes up the complete set of chromosomes in the baby. The billions of building blocks, called base pairs, that make up our chromosomes must come together nearly perfectly for a healthy baby to form. What is most amazing is that this usually happens. Occasionally pieces of chromosomes may be deleted, entire chromosomes can be lost, or extra chromosomes may be added, resulting in disease states. Many of the mental retardation syndromes, such as Down's syndrome (Trisomy 21), are a result of random genetic events. The random chromosomal abnormalities cannot be predicted in advance.

Age alone is a strong risk factor for these random chromosomal mistakes. At age 20 the risk of a chromosomal disorder is low, around one in 500. At 35 years of age that risk has increased to one in 200. By age 49 the risk is about one in ten. *I strongly recommend that all women who will be 35 years or older when the baby is born consider having preconceptional genetic counseling and first trimester screening (early ultrasound and blood testing) and be counseled about amniocentesis (or chorionic villus sampling) and have a more detailed ultrasound in the second trimester.* During amniocentesis, an ultrasound-guided needle is used to remove a small amount of amniotic fluid from the sac of water around the baby; a chorionic villus sampling involves the removal of a small piece of the placenta. Both tests are used to do a chromosomal analysis (called a karyotype), which looks for any evidence of chromosomal (genetic) disorders. You should discuss the choice of which test would be best for you with your physician. In Chapter 10, I will review the relationship between age and genetic problems in greater detail.

ENVIRONMENTAL EXPOSURES

There are literally thousands of chemicals that a woman could potentially be exposed to at work or at home. Many of these chemicals have unknown potential for adverse consequences to the early pregnancy. Some of the better-studied agents with known adverse reproductive effects include alcohol, cigarettes, certain recreational drugs (cocaine, heroin, and marijuana), organic solvents, radiation, lead, mercury, pesticides, and vinyl monomers (used in the manufacture of plastics). Keep in mind that far and away the largest sources of environmental toxins for most people are alcohol, cigarettes, and illicit drugs.

The good news is that it appears many of the chemicals in the environment around us do not have adverse reproductive consequences. Figure 3.6 gives regional phone numbers you can call with questions regarding exposures you might be concerned about, and also shows the names and phone numbers of some of the organizations offering databases. Your local university or medical library may also have a computer database for searching for information on the known risks associated with a chemical. I suggest that if you work with chemicals on the job, you should look at the ingredients and write down the names on a piece of paper. Call or get on-line with one of the sources listed to find out whether anything is known about that particular substance. Also, bring that list with you to your preconceptional counseling visit with your physician.

There are many simple steps you can take to avoid excessive exposure to environmental hazards. For instance, stop drinking alcohol or using recreational drugs before attempting to conceive. If you are using a cleaning solvent or painting, make sure that all the windows are open and a fan is blowing. You can avoid all skin contact with chemicals by wearing rubber gloves and most respiratory contact by using a small respirator mask purchased at a hardware store. Certainly, the best way would be to avoid these chemicals entirely.

My wife and I moved into our new house soon after she became pregnant with our first child. She capitalized on her new pregnancy status by getting me to do all the interior painting so she could avoid the potentially harmful chemicals. I couldn't argue with her reasoning, even though I knew she was glad to have the excuse, since she hates painting.

Figure 3.6

RESOURCES FOR QUESTIONS ABOUT EXPOSURE TO
TERATOGENIC CHEMICALS IN EARLY PREGNANCY

- **If you live east of the Mississippi:**
  Massachusetts Teratogen Information Service
  Boston, Mass.
  (617) 466–8474
- **If you live west of the Mississippi:**
  Pregnancy Riskline
  Salt Lake City, Utah
  (801) 328–2229
- **Grateful Med (Toxline, Toxnet, and Medline)**
  (800) 638–8480
  Access through the National Institutes of Health website at: *www.nih.gov* or through the National Library of Medicine at: *www.igm.nlm.nih.gov*
- **Reprotox**
  (202) 293–5137 (Washington, D.C.)
- **Reprorisk**
  (800) 525–9083
- **Shepherd's Catalog of Teratogenic Agents**
  (206) 543–3373 (Seattle, Wash.)

Certain plants, animals, and nutritional supplements are prone to concentrate toxic substances. This means that you should avoid consuming these, both before and after becoming pregnant. I'll tell you exactly which foods those are and provide specific dietary recommendations in Chapter 7.

SOCIAL, FINANCIAL, AND PSYCHOLOGICAL CONSIDERATIONS

Pregnancy and parenthood are truly life-altering events. There is no way to describe how profoundly the changes will impact your lives. Besides the time and emotional investment, there are also many practical considerations that need to be addressed. You will have to consider the subjects of health insurance, financial planning, and career planning *before you become pregnant*.

Health Insurance

Many employers have a designated period of time that you must be employed before your health insurance will cover a pregnancy. Assuming you are covered, what percentage of the pregnancy will be covered by your plan? What if there is a complication? What are the limits to the coverage? You will need the answers to these questions before getting pregnant so that you aren't surprised by unexpected bills.

What if you are planning to quit your job or have found a better job at another company? In almost all cases, a health insurance company must offer you continued health insurance coverage after you have left a job, as long as you continue to pay the premiums yourself. Eligibility for continued coverage is mandated in most cases by federal guidelines arising from the Consolidated Omnibus Budget Reconciliation Act of 1985, referred

Figure 3.7

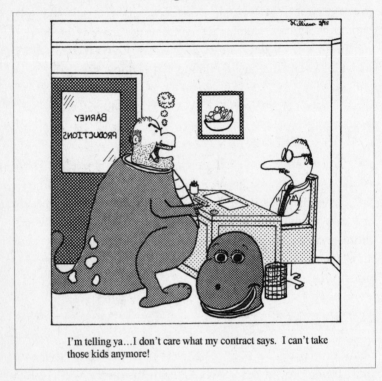

I'm telling ya...I don't care what my contract says. I can't take those kids anymore!

to as COBRA rules. COBRA requires most companies employing 20 or more people to continue offering insurance coverage at a group rate, at your expense, for up to 18 months if:

- Your employment is terminated (except for gross misconduct); or
- Your working hours are reduced so that you're ineligible for group coverage.

Disability, dependents of a deceased employee, divorce or separation, all have different terms. Under federal and most state statutes you usually have 60 days to notify your employer/insurance company of your desire to continue coverage. Do this in writing and make sure to enclose a check for the appropriate amount. It is your responsibility, not the employer's or insurance company's, to contact the appropriate people and pay the correct premium, so don't expect them to come to you. COBRA usually assures a coverage period of 18 months after termination of your previous job; however, it may be longer in some cases. Do not assume anything—*contact your company's human resources department before you leave your job* to make sure you understand all of your options, or lack thereof.

Many states have their own statutes protecting citizens from losing insurance coverage due to job changes. Frequently, state laws take up where the federal government left off, assisting the employees of companies with fewer than 20 full-time employees, or the employees of companies that, for whatever reason, are not required to provide COBRA continuation. Open your phone book and contact your state government for information regarding the specific laws in your state.

If you are considering leaving your job during your pregnancy, contact the human resources department of your company and find out how you can extend your health coverage. Do this before you leave your job! Also, find out if your next employer's health insurance coverage will consider any preexisting medical conditions. You may find that continuing your previous insurance under COBRA would save you money if you were involved in treatment or had a preexisting condition not covered by your future insurance carrier. Don't get caught without coverage, especially if you're planning to get pregnant. If you have a complication, especially a premature infant, the bills can add up to hundreds of thousands of dollars.

Professional Considerations

It would be helpful to find out your company's policies toward pregnancy and maternity leave in advance. You should also find out how your company handles employees with complications during the pregnancy, especially if the complication would require you to be out of work for a prolonged period of time. Does the future father's company offer paternity leave?

My wife and I had many discussions about what she would do about her job after the birth of our first child. Go back to work after the six weeks of maternity leave? Be part-time at work for a while? Day care? A nanny? Be a stay-at-home mom for a while and then go back? Some couples may consider the husband's job to be more flexible, and then the husband will have to deal with these same issues. In any case, any choice you make, other than returning immediately after maternity leave, can have negative consequences on your career goals.

This issue of professional goals versus family responsibilities has grown far more complicated as women professionals become increasingly integrated into the business world. Many women are delaying their childbearing for years in order to firmly establish their professional positions before starting their family. *I recommend that all couples spend time talking about how they will deal with the daily care of the child, before getting pregnant.* This allows each partner to think about the issues without the pressure of the deadline of your due date.

Financial Considerations

No couple has ever said "Having a baby was a lot cheaper than we thought it would be." If you don't have medical insurance, or your insurance only pays a fraction of the total bills (many insurers cover 70 or 80 percent), then you will need to know how much having a baby will cost. The average cost of prenatal care and delivery in the United States is nearly $10,000, and if you have twins the average cost will be over $30,000. It is estimated that it will cost over $300,000 to raise a child from birth to age 18. I was dumbfounded by the amount of money we spent preparing for the arrival of our first baby, much less the cost of raising a child for 18 years! Talk to friends and family who have recently had a baby to get a general estimate of the costs involved. At least you will know what to expect, and it may decrease some of the inevitable arguments with your spouse about how much money is being spent preparing for the new addition to the family.

Figure 3.8

SUMMARY

Nutrition

- All women of childbearing age should take one prenatal multivitamin that meets but does not exceed the recommended daily allowances of all vitamins and minerals and contains 0.4 to 0.6 milligrams (400 to 600 micrograms) of folic acid in each tablet, beginning at least one month prior to conception.
- If taking oral contraceptives up until the cycle of conception, increase dose of folic acid to 1.0 milligrams each day, beginning at least one month prior to conception.
- If you have previously had a child affected with a neural tube defect, discuss this with your physician. In this circumstance the recommended daily dose of folic acid is 4.0 milligrams each day, beginning at least one month

prior to conception. *Do not take more than one prenatal multivitamin per day.* You will need a separate supplement of folic acid in addition to your daily prenatal multivitamin.

- If a parent, sibling, or other close relative has been affected with a neural tube defect, discuss the correct dose of folic acid with your physician.

Immunizations/Infections
Prior to conception see your physician to test for:
- *Strongly recommended*
  Rubella/Varicella (chicken pox)—immunize if negative three months prior to conceiving
  Bacterial vaginosis—screening and treatment with antibiotics if infected
- *Suggested (even if not at risk)*
  HIV/Syphilis/Gonorrhea/Chlamydia
- *If in a risk group*
  Toxoplasmosis/Tuberculosis/Cytomegalovirus

Medications/Medical Problems
- Discuss all chronic medications or medical problems with your physician prior to pregnancy.

Genetic Counseling
- All women more than 35 years old should be offered preconceptional genetic counseling by a physician or genetics counselor.
- Regardless of age, all couples with family histories of inherited diseases should be seen by a physician or genetics counselor prior to pregnancy.
- At-risk couples should discuss options for testing, treatment, and lifestyle changes before becoming pregnant.

Environmental Exposures

- Contact the agencies in Figure 3.6 to learn more about the effects of any environmental exposures on conception or pregnancy.

Social Considerations

- Both the male and female partner should review all the details of their health insurance as it relates to pregnancy and labor before becoming pregnant.
- Familiarize yourself with your company's maternity (or paternity) leave policy before the pregnancy.
- Sit down with your partner and discuss the financial, professional, and personal changes that will take place after the baby is born.

4

Stopping Birth Control

SINCE the 1970s, contraception has become very common and well accepted by Americans. Ease of access to effective birth-control methods has enabled women to assume better control of their reproductive destinies. The ability to plan and avoid pregnancies has played a key role in allowing women to pursue higher education and professional careers.

The focus of this chapter is to learn about the fertility-reducing effects of some forms of birth control and to show you how to avoid any contraceptive-related delays in becoming pregnant. Some contraceptive methods can significantly reduce your chances of conceiving for a prolonged period after the last dose of medication. Depo-Provera (Upjohn) can cause the most profound reduction in fertility, lasting as long as nine months after the last dose. Other hormonal contraceptive methods, such as estrogen and progestin combinations (oral contraceptives, NUVA ring, EVRA patch), implantable devices (Norplant System, Jadelle, and Implanon), and the progestin-containing intrauterine device (IUD) (Mirena), can also prolong the time it takes to become pregnant. For this reason, I will now discuss the best time to discontinue a birth-control method if you want to maximize your chances of becoming pregnant as quickly as possible.

ORAL CONTRACEPTIVES

When we began planning for our first child, my wife asked me when she should stop her birth-control pills. Because an estimated 15 million American women use birth-control pills, this is an important and commonly asked question. The answer is fairly straightforward for most women, but there are some subtleties that may apply to your own situation. Duration of use, previous history of irregular periods before starting oral contraceptives, any significant change in weight or activity level since beginning the pills, and some other less common factors may alter the recommendations.

Decreased Fertility Following Oral Contraceptive Use

There is no evidence or reason to think that oral contraceptives cause infertility after they have been stopped. There is evidence, however, that a period of decreased fertility may follow the use of oral contraceptives. A number of studies have evaluated this reduction in fertility following the use of birth control pills. Drs. S. Harlap and M. Baras from Hadassah Medical School in Israel published a study in the *International Journal of Fertility* that examined the histories of women who used oral contraceptives and then stopped them with the intention to conceive. They showed that these women had a 30 percent smaller chance of conceiving during the first month after stopping the pills. The reduction in fertility disappeared after three months. This doesn't sound like such a big deal, but the issue turns out to be more complicated.

A study in the journal *Fertility and Sterility* by Dr. Michael Bracken and colleagues at Yale University showed that for women using oral contraceptives (at the dosage commonly prescribed in the United States), compared to women using other forms of birth control, there was about a one-month delay in the average time it took to get pregnant. The average time for women who were not previously on the pill was three months, while previous oral contraceptive users took four months to conceive. The researchers also showed that in the first cycle the probability of conception was about 24 percent for oral contraceptive users, but 35 percent for all others. This represents about a one-third reduction in conception rates for women in the first month following use of oral contraceptives. Most importantly, and to the surprise of the investigators, they found that this one-third-lower chance of conceiving per monthly cycle continued for at least one year.

This study showed a significant decrease in conception rates for the first month after discontinuing oral contraceptives. Additionally, while the average time to become pregnant may only differ by about one month, in a minority of women there can be a prolonged delay. For these women, the residual effects of oral contraceptive use may result in a reduction in fertility that persists for a year or possibly longer.

I have many patients who report a delay in the return of their menstrual cycles after oral contraceptive use. Doctors refer to this as post-pill amenorrhea. There is some controversy as to whether this limited absence of the menstrual periods, after discontinuing use of oral contraceptives, has any significance. It has been difficult to determine if this phenomenon is actually related to the pills or if it's due to previous or acquired problems with the menstrual cycles or if it's merely a coincidence.

In general, if you want to maximize your chances of becoming pregnant on the first attempt, *you should discontinue your oral contraceptives two to three months before attempting to conceive.* Of course, this means you must use a barrier form of contraception in the interim so you won't get pregnant earlier than desired.

Changes in Weight or Activity Level While Taking Oral Contraceptives or Previous History of Abnormal Menstrual Cycles

Oral contraceptives effectively mask menstrual irregularities by producing artificially normal cycles. Many women assume that everything is normal with their menstrual cycles while they're taking oral contraceptives. Whether or not your menstrual cycles return normally could depend on many factors: previous menstrual regularity, duration of oral contraceptive use, medical problems, and activity level and/or weight changes while on the pills. Certainly, *if you had irregular periods before starting the oral contraceptives, or if you were placed on the pill to regulate your cycle, you will want to stop the medication at least three to six months prior to your attempts to conceive.* If your cycles were irregular before the oral contraceptives, then chances are they will be equally irregular after stopping them.

After you stop taking your pills, if you have gone three months without having a period you should consult your physician for help. During the first cycle after stopping the pills you may not ovulate when you would expect to, so if you don't want to get pregnant yet you should use condoms or another barrier form of birth control. You may also want to use a home ovulation-prediction kit or basal-body-temperature chart to see if and when you ovulate (see instructions in Chapter 5).

Many women's menstrual cycles are quite sensitive to weight changes, either weight gain or loss (see Chapter 6). With even a 5 to 10 percent increase in body weight, some women will develop irregular periods. It is very common for my patients to report that they started birth-control pills during high school or in college. They come to see me in their late twenties or early thirties, planning to become pregnant. Not surprisingly, most of these women are more than 5 percent heavier than they were in college. I think the majority of both men and women would fall into that category—I certainly do. I counsel this group of women to *stop using the oral contraceptives at least three or four months before trying to conceive, in case the additional weight has made their menstrual cycles irregular.*

On the other hand, a significant weight loss can also make your cycles irregular. Prior to our attempts to conceive, my wife, Kara, was taking oral contraceptives and also running marathons, so she had lost a significant amount of weight while on the pill. There were two issues we had to resolve with her specific situation: the first was the fact that women who exercise intensely tend to have irregular menstrual cycles, and the second was that she had decreased her weight significantly

Figure 4.1
RELATIONSHIP BETWEEN WEIGHT AND FERTILITY

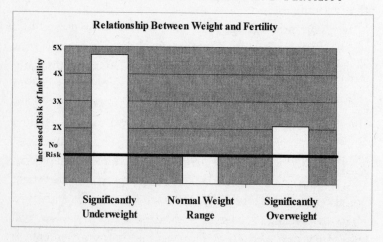

B.B. Green, N.S. Weiss, and J.R. Daling. "Risk of Ovulatory Infertility in Relation to Body Weight." *Fertility and Sterility* 50 (1988): 721–26. Copyright © 1988, Elsevier Science.

while on the oral contraceptives. Both the intense exercise and the weight loss could make her cycles irregular or nonexistent, though the pills kept her cycles artificially regular. There was a good chance that Kara would have irregular cycles when she stopped taking the pill.

Ultimately, we decided that Kara would increase her weight by about six or seven pounds to reestablish her previous weight but continue to use the birth-control pills until two months before trying to conceive. We hoped that by putting on a little body fat Kara would have normal menstrual cycles after stopping the use of oral contraceptives. Fortunately her fertility was not impaired, and we conceived quickly. (For a detailed look at weight, exercise, body fat, and fertility, see Chapter 6.)

Duration of Oral Contraceptive Use

Marie, 30, came in to see me when she stopped menstruating. She had been on oral contraceptives for nine years and had progressively lighter and shorter menstrual cycles until they had ceased altogether. We did a basic evaluation, including a pregnancy test, which was negative. I explained to her that an estimated 5 percent of women (one in 20) will stop having menstrual periods if they stay on oral contraceptives for many years. She was satisfied with that answer, but then she asked me if I thought this would impact her ability to become pregnant. She and her husband were planning to conceive in about six months.

A few studies have evaluated the relationship between long-term use of oral contraceptives and fertility. If you have been on oral contraceptives for a long time, the lining of the uterus tends to become atrophic, or very thin. Additionally, the brain and ovaries, which control the menstrual cycle, have been suppressed for a prolonged period. It makes sense that the longer you are on the pill, the more likely you will have reduced fertility after discontinuing the medication.

Some investigators believe there is a demonstrable difference between women who have used oral contraceptives for two years or less and those who have been on the pill for longer than two years. Although this isn't certain, I think it reasonable to suggest that the longer you have been on the pill, the more you should consider leaving a comfortable "cushion" before trying to conceive. For most women on oral contraceptives, three months should suffice. However, *if you have been taking the pill for longer than two years, or previously had abnormal cycles, stop three to six months in advance of your attempts to conceive* if you want to maximize your chances of getting pregnant as quickly as possible.

Oral Contraceptives and Birth Defects

There is no evidence and no reason to think that using birth-control pills up until the cycle of conception has any direct relationship with birth defects. However, *oral contraceptives can decrease the amount of many vitamins and minerals in your body despite appropriate levels of supplementation. This has been verified with vitamins C, B_1, B_2, B_6, B_{12}, folic acid, magnesium, calcium, and zinc.* Particularly important for women attempting to conceive is the decrease in blood levels of folic acid when taking oral contraceptives. All women who could potentially become pregnant are encouraged to take 0.4 milligrams of folic acid each day in order to decrease the risk of birth defects involving the brain and spinal cord (see Chapter 3). But *if you are taking oral contraceptives up until the time* *you are going to try to get pregnant, you should take 0.8 to 1.0 milligrams of folic acid per day,* rather than the 0.4 milligrams normally recommended.

The only known direct effect I am aware of from continuing oral contraceptives until the cycle of conception is a very small increased chance of having twins with that first cycle. The increase in the rate of twins is so small that I hesitate to include the information, because I don't think it is necessary for couples to factor it into the decision-making process.

DEPO-PROVERA

Depo-Provera (Upjohn), commonly called Depo, is an injectable form of birth control that has waned in popularity due to concerns about bone density with chronic use. The active ingredient is a type of hormone called a progestin (medroxyprogesterone acetate). The Depo-Provera shot is given every twelve weeks and is a reliable form of birth control. As you would expect, the medication does not wear off completely after three months of use. In most women, after 12 to 14 weeks the contraceptive action starts to become less reliable. In reality, the delay to conception can be as much as nine months following the last injection. This is not to say that you cannot get pregnant for nine months, but rather that your chances can be significantly reduced.

Tammy, 28, had received a Depo shot the previous month, but then decided she wanted to become pregnant. She came to me specifically to ask if there was some way to get the medication out of her system faster so she could conceive. I told her that unfortunately I had no suggestions. She returned six months later pregnant and ready to start her prenatal care.

The duration of use does not seem to increase this nine-month delay. There is no permanent decrease in fertility associated with the use of Depo-Provera. Keep in mind that if you have a strict timetable for the pregnancy, *do not receive a shot within one year in advance of your attempts at getting pregnant.*

NORPLANT

The Norplant System (Wyeth-Ayerst) involves the insertion of six matchstick-size silastic implants under the skin in the upper arm. The implants slowly release one of the progestational hormones (levonorgestrel) into the surrounding tissue, which then absorbs the hormones into the bloodstream. The Norplant lasts for five years and is a reliable form of birth control. In 2002 Norplant was taken off the market, but women may still have the Norplant in place. By the end of 2007 it would be expected that all women will have had their implants removed.

Unlike oral contraceptives or Depo-Provera, Norplant appears to allow a more rapid return to fertility. Studies have shown that conception rates rapidly return to normal levels after removal and do not seem to be associated with duration of use. However, the Norplant causes a thinning of the uterine lining, *so you should still discontinue its use at least a month or two before attempting to conceive.*

Jadelle is another implantable device that is sometimes referred to as "Norplant 2." It involves only two rods that contain levonorgestrel, the same medication as Norplant. Jadelle lasts for five years. It is available in Europe, and it is uncertain whether it will be marketed in the U.S.

INTRAUTERINE DEVICE (IUD)

The IUD is a very effective form of birth control. It is a small, T-shaped plastic device that is placed in the uterine cavity. There are two types of IUDs currently in use in the United States: the copper IUD and the progestin IUD.

The IUD works in various ways, but a major mechanism of action of the copper IUD in preventing conception is by causing a low-grade inflammation in the uterine lining and Fallopian tubes, which inactivates the sperm as they pass through on their way to find the egg. Additionally, the low-grade inflammation may have a further contraceptive effect should the egg become fertilized, since the inflamed uterine lining is very inhospitable to implantation of the embryo. In the United States, the copper IUD is approved for up to ten years of use before removal. The progestin IUD slowly releases the synthetic hormone medroxyprogesterone acetate over five years. This IUD not only irritates the uterine lining, but the progestin also makes the lining very thin (atrophic). This combination of inflammation and atrophy of the uterine lining results in an effective contraceptive for five years.

The inflammation and/or thinning of the uterine lining should resolve soon after the removal of the IUD. It is prudent to allow a month or two after the use of either type of IUD before trying to get pregnant.

The IUD is the only contraceptive method associated with a higher risk of permanent infertility. A serious bacterial infection from an organism called *Actinomyces* has been associated with IUD use, albeit only rarely. The organism can cause a pelvic infection that may result in tubal or ovarian scarring and subsequent infertility. Fortunately, this is a very rare occurrence.

IMPLANON

The newest form of birth control available is a single implant called Implanon. Similar to Norplant or Jadelle, the contraceptive device is inserted under the skin of the upper arm. The medication contained within the single rod is called etonogestrel, a type of progestin. Implanon lasts for three years. The return to normal fertility following removal should be fairly rapid. My recommendation is to discontinue Implanon at least one or two months prior to the time you want to start trying to get pregnant.

BARRIER FORMS OF CONTRACEPTION

The remainder of birth-control methods are mostly barrier forms such as the condom, diaphragm, sponge, spermicidal jelly, and cervical cap. These nonhormonal methods do not cause decreased fertility or infertility, and therefore require no special recommendations.

Figure 4.2
SUMMARY

Oral Contraceptives ("The Pill")	1. If you have taken the pill for less than two years, stop two to three months before attempting to conceive.
	2. If you have taken the pill for more than two years, stop three to six months before attempting to conceive.
	3. If you experienced menstrual irregularities before starting the pill, stop at

Figure 4.2 (continued)

Oral Contraceptives ("The Pill") *continued*	least three to six months before attempting to conceive to identify any potential problems. 4. If you plan to take the pill up until the time you will begin trying to conceive, then take a prenatal multivitamin but also take an extra 400 micrograms (0.4 milligrams) of folic acid (by separate supplement) to give you a total of 800 micrograms (0.8 milligrams) to 1 milligram daily. 5. Consider any change in weight or exercise that may have occurred since you started taking the pill. These factors may affect your menstrual cycle regularity after stopping the pill (see Chapter 6).
Depo-Provera (Depo)	Do not receive a Depo-Provera shot within one year of attempting to conceive.
Norplant, Implanon, Jadelle	Have any implant removed at least two months before attempting to conceive.
Intrauterine Device (IUD)	Have the IUD removed at least two months before attempting to conceive.

5

—

Timing Is Everything: Predicting Ovulation

> Observe due measure, for right timing is in all
> things the most important fact.
>
> —*Hesiod,* Works and Days, *700 B.C.*

FOR most couples, being able to accurately predict
ovulation is the single most important factor in getting pregnant quickly. This chapter will review all you need to know
about ovulation prediction to allow you to conceive as quickly
as possible. If a healthy, fertile couple can accurately pinpoint
their day of ovulation and time their sexual intercourse to coincide with it, they should significantly decrease the time it
takes to conceive a healthy baby.

THE 14-DAY FALLACY

Ovulation is the medical term for the release of the egg from
the ovary. While sperm can survive and continue to fertilize an
egg for 48 to 72 hours (two to three days) after intercourse, the

egg can only survive for 12 to 24 hours after ovulation. This creates a narrow window of opportunity for fertilization. In order to time your intercourse appropriately, it is necessary to predict your ovulation reliably. *In fertile couples, incorrect timing of intercourse is the most common cause of prolonging the time to conception.*

Working in a university community, I see many married undergraduate and graduate students, as well as professors, who are planning to get pregnant soon or who have been trying for a few months and are discouraged at not becoming pregnant. These couples have a strict timetable. They need to plan their delivery during the summer months so it does not interfere with their busy schedules during the school year.

Nearly all of these well-educated patients have read somewhere or been told that women ovulate around day 14 of their menstrual cycle, so they should concentrate their intercourse around those days. They are surprised when I tell them that "normal" women may ovulate as much as five days before or one week after that day. When these couples substitute a reliable method of ovulation prediction for the "14-day rule," they are far more successful at conceiving a healthy child in the timeframe they need to fit their careers.

As we reviewed in Chapter 1, the first day of bleeding is the first day of the menstrual cycle. What is relatively fixed about the menstrual cycle is that ovulation usually occurs about 14 days before the last day of a woman's menstrual cycle, the day before her menstrual bleeding begins. Therefore, the preovulation period of the menstrual cycle can vary substantially. Because the average length of a menstrual cycle is 28 days, the commonly quoted day of ovulation is cycle day 14 (subtract 14 days from a 28-day cycle). Many couples hear from their doctors or other sources that the fastest way to get pregnant is to concentrate sexual intercourse around the fourteenth day of the woman's menstrual cycle.

Most women, however, do not have the average 28-day cycle and may have a cycle length between 23 and 35 days. Therefore, in women with menstrual cycles considered to be of normal length (every 23 to 35 days), *ovulation can occur anywhere between cycle day 9 (for a 23-day cycle) and cycle day 21 (for a 35-day cycle)*. A lot of readers are probably saying at this point, "I'm normal after all!" This misconception about what is a normal menstrual cycle is very common.

This significant variation in the length of the woman's menstrual cycle is the reason why the "14-day rule" will not

Figure 5.1

VARIATIONS IN THE MENSTRUAL CYCLE

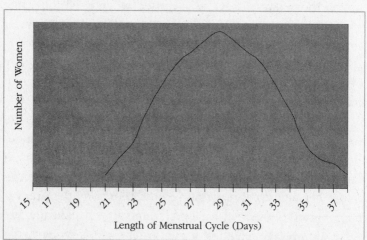

The exact middle of the curve falls on 28 days. This is the average cycle length. But the vast majority of women do *not* have cycles that are 28 days in length. For women whose cycles are longer or shorter than 28 days, it is unlikely that their ovulation will fall on day 14.

necessarily maximize your chances of getting pregnant quickly. To further complicate matters, the body is not a clock, and you may not ovulate on the same cycle day from month to month.

During the time I was writing this book I found out from one of my sisters-in-law that she and her husband had been trying to get pregnant without success for nine months. During our conversation, she indicated that she had a 35-day menstrual cycle, and they had not been using any ovulation-prediction method. They had been concentrating their intercourse during the "most fertile time"—the days around cycle day 14. I explained that with a 35-day menstrual cycle she probably wasn't ovulating until as late as cycle day 21, and this was probably why they had not become pregnant. I mailed them a coupon for an ovulation-prediction kit to use with her next cycle. The kit became positive on cycle day 19, they had intercourse that day and the following day, and got pregnant that month.

HOW OVULATION OCCURS

You now know that you can't assume your ovulation falls on any given cycle day. You need to find a way to predict the day when your ovulation will occur. In order to do that, it will help you to know what ovulation is, what's going on in your body when you ovulate, and what the signs of ovulation are.

During the first week of the menstrual cycle, the body selects one egg to be released from an ovary that month. As you saw in Chapter 1, the woman's body has two ovaries, either one of which can generate the egg in any given month. The process of releasing the egg and preparing the woman's body for possible pregnancy is dominated by four hormones: *estrogen, luteinizing hormone (LH), follicle stimulating hormone (FSH), and progesterone*. Tests that predict ovulation either measure the amount of one or more of these hormones or test for the characteristic signs they produce in a woman's body.

Estrogen, stimulated by FSH released from the brain, is the first hormone to control the events of the woman's menstrual cycle. This hormone is produced in the ovary by cells surrounding the egg that has been selected for release. During the first half of the menstrual cycle, estrogen levels rise continually.

The increased estrogen level promotes the growth of a thick uterine lining, which will help the fertilized egg implant and grow in the uterus. Estrogen also changes the consistency and quantity of the cervical mucus—as estrogen levels rise, the mucus becomes increasingly slippery, transparent, and abundant. This serves as the basis for the cervical mucus method of ovulation prediction.

Shortly after the peak of the estrogen rise, the brain releases LH into the bloodstream. The LH is not released all at once but rather rises and then falls over a 24- to 48-hour period. The surge of LH usually occurs around the middle of the cycle, but as we just reviewed, this can vary, depending on the length of each woman's cycle. It's also important to remember that the release of LH may not occur on exactly the same day of each cycle.

The onset of the LH rise in blood most commonly occurs during the early morning hours (between 3 and 5 A.M.). The kidneys filter the blood and remove the LH from the system over four to six hours, depositing the LH in the urine. This is why ovulation-prediction kits, which measure LH levels in the urine, work better when you *don't* use your first morning urine to conduct the test—because the LH may not be concentrated in the urine yet.

Sleep cycles probably also influence the timing of LH release. Women with irregular sleep patterns, or "graveyard shift" workers, may be more likely to surge in the afternoon while they are asleep.

When the LH is released, it courses through the bloodstream to the ovary. Once there, it triggers the ovary to release proteins called enzymes. These enzymes create a hole in the wall of the small sac, or follicle, that holds the egg selected for that cycle. Through this opening in the follicle, the egg and the surrounding fluid pour out. This leaking of the egg and fluid from the ovary is called *ovulation*.

The released egg moves into the Fallopian tube, where fertilization by the sperm usually takes place. *The time from the beginning of the LH rise to the moment of ovulation is about 36 hours.*

The remaining empty follicle, from which the egg was released, then re-forms and becomes the corpus luteum. It is the

Figure 5.2

HORMONAL CHANGES DURING A
28-DAY MENSTRUAL CYCLE

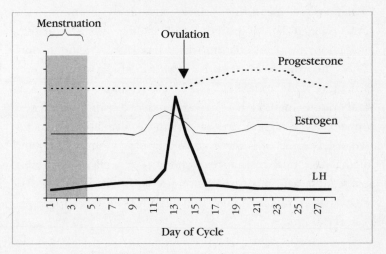

corpus luteum that releases the hormone progesterone following ovulation. Progesterone dominates the second half of the menstrual cycle. Rising levels of progesterone cause a woman's core body temperature to rise significantly. This temperature change serves as the basis for the basal body temperature (BBT) method of predicting ovulation.

Using hormonal and other changes in a woman's body over the course of a menstrual cycle, physicians and other experts have devised various methods for predicting ovulation. Many of these methods can be used at home, including:

- Measuring luteinizing hormone (LH) and/or estrogen levels in the urine;
- Following changes in body temperature;
- Noting changes in the appearance of cervical mucus;
- Recognizing the pain associated with ovulation;
- Monitoring changes in salivary and cervical-mucus electrical resistance.

Of these, the two most common methods for predicting ovulation are measuring urinary luteinizing hormone (LH) levels, which is the marker used by the home ovulation-prediction kits, and charting daily basal body temperatures. With the mass marketing of affordable and accurate ovulation-prediction kits, the less reliable basal-body-temperature method has become much less popular. There are also two high-technology methods available for home ovulation prediction—computerized urinary monitors and oral/vaginal electrical resistance monitors—as well as two other less reliable methods of ovulation prediction: recognizing ovulatory pain (*"mittelschmerz"*) and changes in the appearance of cervical mucus.

OVULATION-PREDICTION KITS

The use of ovulation-prediction kits has grown dramatically in the past few years, as has the number of companies selling these kits. This popularity is due to the accuracy of these kits, their reasonable price, and the ease of performing the test in the privacy of your own home. However, ovulation-prediction kits are still a source of confusion and frustration for many couples. Questions about the proper use of the kits are a common reason for patients calling our clinic. Although I highly recommend using these kits, they are still not completely user-friendly. The information below should help simplify the use of these kits and help them to be as accurate as possible. Most important is to make sure that you read the instructions for the kit you purchase to make sure you are using and interpreting it correctly.

How Ovulation-Prediction Kits Work

Because LH is the hormone measured by the ovulation-prediction kits, these kits are more accurately described as LH detection kits. You may see them labeled in the drugstore with either name. The ovulation-prediction kits use special chemicals to recognize the presence of LH in a small sample of urine. Three drops of urine placed in one end of a test cassette are enough to determine whether LH is present in significant amounts in the urine. If your test is positive, you know that your LH is rising and the egg will be released soon.

Some of my patients think they will save some money by spacing out their tests to every two days instead of every 24 hours. But as I described above, *the recognizable LH rise may only last 24 hours, so if you wait two days between tests you may miss this crucial moment in your cycle.* Once you have started your testing, you should continue to do it daily—at about the same time every day. If you check your urine at about the same time every day, you should not miss the LH rise.

It is possible that when you test your urine the LH surge has just occurred, resulting in a positive test result. Or it may be that the LH surge is about to occur, so your test kit still shows a negative result. Therefore, a positive result could mean that the LH rise just occurred and the egg will not be released for up to 40 hours or that the LH rise occurred 24 hours ago and the egg may be released very soon.

Although this may seem like a somewhat inexact prediction, as long as you have intercourse on the day of a positive result from your kit, and more importantly, again 24 hours later, you should cover all possibilities. I also recommend having intercourse a third time, the second day after a positive result, although this is less crucial. If you want to be more exact but also spend more money, you can use ovulation-prediction kits every 12 hours. This will better define the beginning of the LH surge and increase the ability of the kits to recognize the rise in LH to more than 95 percent accuracy.

How to Obtain a Kit

Ovulation-prediction kits can be purchased from any local pharmacy or through 1-800 telephone numbers for home delivery. The kits come with 5, 6, 9, or 10 days of tests included and cost between $25 and $40, depending on how many days of tests are included.

I am frequently asked which kits are the most accurate. There is limited information on the comparison of kits. One unpublished study in 1997, by Dr. D. S. Wickman, Dr. P. B. Miller, and Dr. M. R. Soules at the University of Washington

School of Medicine, compared OvuQuick, OvuQuick One-Step, Clearplan Easy, SureStep, and EZ-LH brands. The three best performers were OvuQuick, OvuQuick One-Step, and Clearplan Easy. Each of these three best-performing kits had about 90 percent accuracy when used once a day and approached 100 percent accuracy when a test was used every 12 hours (twice a day). Since this study there have been many new brands introduced to the market, and it is uncertain how they compare to one another in terms of accuracy.

When Should I Start Using the Test Kit?

Because the ovulation-prediction kits include only 5 to 10 test cassettes per kit, you do not want to begin testing too early and run out of tests before your LH rises. Therefore, you need to make a reasonable guess as to the length of your menstrual cycle. In Figure 5.3, I have provided an easy-to-reference chart that shows you what day to start your urinary testing depending on the length of your cycles. It is important that you start testing your urine at least a few days before the expected day of the LH rise. Besides the fact that you should not start testing too late in the cycle and miss the LH rise, it will be beneficial to have a few days of negative test results so that you have something to compare with the positive one.

If your cycles are between 21 and 32 days in length you probably only need to buy a 5- or 6-day kit. If your cycle is greater than 32 days I recommend that you purchase one of the 9- or 10-day kits (or be prepared to buy a second 5-day kit if you haven't seen a positive result from your first kit). Once you have used the longer kit for a cycle and discovered what day you ovulate, then you can probably switch to the shorter-duration kits. *Remember that the body is not a clock and you may not ovulate on the same day each month*.

Figure 5.3

WHEN TO START TESTING YOUR LH LEVEL

SUGGESTED KIT LENGTH	AVERAGE CYCLE LENGTH	DAY OF CYCLE TO BEGIN TESTING
5- or 6-Day Kit	21 days	day 6
	22 days	day 6
	23 days	day 7
	24 days	day 8
	25 days	day 9
	26 days	day 10
	27 days	day 10
	28 days	day 11
	29 days	day 11
	30 days	day 12
	31 days	day 12
	32 days	day 13
9- or 10-Day Kit	33 days	day 13
	34 days	day 14
	35 days	day 14

What's the Best Time of Day to Perform the Test?

Most package inserts in the kits tell you that the best time to do a test is between 10 A.M. and 8 P.M. The study I mentioned earlier, by Drs. Wickman, Miller, and Soules, indicated that testing in the morning was consistently about 10 percent more accurate than testing in the evening. Optimally, late morning is probably the best time to test; however, many women who work outside the home do not want to bring a test to work with them.

Realistically, you can perform the test in the bathroom stall in exactly five minutes, and no one will be the wiser. For those with a busy schedule or who don't think it would be practical to test at work, I recommend that you test as soon as you get home from work. If you think you might have to work late, always keep an extra test kit in your purse. It's also best not to drink for a few hours before taking the test, so that your urine is maximally concentrated. For my wife, Kara, the best time to test was before lunchtime at work. It wasn't too late in the day, and she usually hadn't had anything to drink since breakfast.

Occasionally I have patients who work nights and report difficulty detecting the LH rise. For my patients who have irregular sleep patterns or who work night shifts, I recommend doing ovulation-prediction kits every 12 hours. Since the LH release is related to sleep cycles, this will help reduce the chances of missing the rise in LH.

Figure 5.4 shows how to read the result of the most common type of ovulation-prediction kits. The test result depends on the comparison of two lines on the test kit; the result is positive if the testing line (the "T" line) is darker than the reference line (the "R" line, also referred to as the "C" line for control). Some of my patients have a difficult time comparing the two lines to determine which is darker. There is another, more user-friendly type of ovulation-prediction kit in which just the appearance of a second line is an indication of a positive result. No comparison of lines is necessary. Another form of the kit allows you to urinate directly on the end of the testing stick so that no collection of urine is required. Make sure to check the specific instructions for the kit you purchase to make sure you are using and interpreting it correctly.

What If I Never Get a Positive Test?

There are a few possible reasons why you may not see a positive test result during a cycle:

Figure 5.4

URINARY OVULATION TEST KIT RESULTS

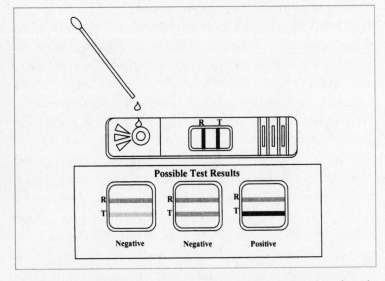

Possible Test Results

R	R	R
T	T	T
Negative	Negative	Positive

In most ovulation-prediction kits there are two letters printed on the side of a large rectangular well, labeled the "C" and the "T." The "C" indicates the "control" band and the "T" indicates the "test" band. Some kits use an "R" (for "reference") band instead of a "C," but they represent the same thing. For the test kit to be working properly, the "C" (or "R") band should appear every time. If no line appears for the "C" band, regardless of whether any line formed at the "T" band, this indicates a faulty test and the results are void. *If the "T" band appears, in most kits it is only considered to be a positive test result if the "T" band is darker than the "C" (or "R") band.*

- The test was used too early or too late in the cycle. If you suspect you may have started too late or ended the testing too early, consider purchasing the 9- or 10-day kit next cycle (if you didn't during the previous cycle). Also review Figure 5.3 to make sure you started the test on the optimal day for your cycle length. This is most commonly a problem for women with long menstrual cycles. If you have a long cycle, don't get frustrated. Continue testing, the positive result may be right around the corner.

- The kit was used incorrectly—user error. If you follow the instructions in the package insert of your kit (and my review above) this should rarely occur. The most common mistakes involve comparing the bands on the kit. If you are uncertain about a result, ask someone else to look at the result and tell you what they see. If you're still unsure, repeat the test a few hours later.

- The kit did not detect the LH surge that actually did occur—product error. Most of the over-the-counter kits are very good, so this should only happen in about one out of ten kits used. As I mentioned, you can do a test kit every 12 hours to increase the accuracy to more than 95 percent, but that is probably not necessary in most cases.

- No LH surge occurred (you did not ovulate). You will probably not be able to distinguish this possibility from the others initially. Every woman has an occasional menstrual cycle when ovulation doesn't occur. However, when ovulation does not occur, menstrual bleeding will not usually begin at the expected time. This delay in bleeding often makes a woman hopeful that she is pregnant but disappointment follows when the result of a pregnancy test is negative.

It is not uncommon for normal women to occasionally have a cycle without ovulating, which results in a significant delay in the onset of menstrual bleeding or irregular bleeding. If this is more than a rare occurrence, you may want to consult your physician. There are many diverse causes for irregular patterns of ovulation and menstrual bleeding, and you will probably benefit from an evaluation by your physician for advice and possibly testing.

Should He Try to "Save Up"?

Many of my patients ask if their husbands should abstain and "save up" the sperm during the first half of the menstrual cycle to improve their chances of conceiving. Unfortunately, abstaining will not result in Superman-like sperm numbers. Having intercourse every 36 to 48 hours should not decrease his sperm count. This also ensures that there is always viable sperm in the female genital tract and is therefore the optimal frequency. The male partner will probably be happy to hear that he shouldn't abstain for prolonged periods of time.

When to Have Sex (If You Are Using an Ovulation-Prediction Kit)

When you begin your ovulation prediction tests (see Figure 5.3), you should have sex about every 36 to 48 hours until you see a positive test result. Once you have a positive ovulation-prediction test, you should have sex that day and again about 24 hours later. As I mentioned earlier, as long as you have intercourse the day of your positive test and the day after, you will maximize your chances for success. If you want to have sex a third time—the following day (two days after a positive test)—that is a good idea but probably not as important. On these days, have sex a single time on each day and space the intercourse 24 hours apart.

Using Ovulation-Prediction Kits

- Count your menstrual cycle *starting from the first day of menstrual bleeding as day 1 of the cycle*.
- Use Figure 5.3 to determine what day to start using the ovulation-prediction kits.

- Once you have started testing, *use the test every day*.
- Take the test at the same time every day. *Don't use your first morning urine to test*. Late morning is probably the best time to test.
- Read the test results at exactly the specified time interval (usually five minutes).
- *Every time you perform a test*, the control or "C" band (sometimes referred to as the "R" band) should form a line. This confirms that the test is working.
- *If the "T" band appears, for most brands of kits it is only considered to be a positive result if the "T" band is darker than the "C" or "R" band*. If they are the same color or if the "T" band is lighter in color, it is a negative result. There are a few brands of test kits that show a positive result merely by any line at all forming at the "T" band. If you have trouble comparing the lines to determine a positive result you may want to purchase one of these easier-to-read brands where a comparison of the bands is not necessary.
- Have sexual intercourse every 36 to 48 hours until you see a positive test result.
- *Have intercourse the day of a positive test and the following day*. You can have intercourse a third time two days after a positive test, but that is probably not as crucial. *Space the intercourse 24 hours apart once your test is positive*.

BASAL-BODY-TEMPERATURE (BBT) CHARTS

The BBT chart has been frustrating patients and physicians for decades because of the difficulty of interpreting it. Basal-body-temperature charts were the mainstay for ovulation prediction for decades until the recent mass marketing of the ovulation-prediction kits. They are still quite popular, and I am frequently asked by patients to interpret their BBT charts during appointments.

The BBT chart's ability to predict ovulation is based on the fact that a woman's body temperature drops subtly at the time of her LH rise (usually very hard to notice), and then goes up significantly over the course of the next few days, staying elevated until the end of her cycle. This rise in temperature is caused by the rising levels of the hormone progesterone produced soon after ovulation. This rise in temperature is the sign that ovulation has occurred.

The main problem with the use of BBT charts for ovulation prediction is that a woman's drop in temperature (at the time of the LH rise) is usually subtle and frequently not recognized until it is compared to the subsequent rise in temperature a few days later. Women often have trouble recognizing the BBT rise until more than 24 hours after ovulation, at which point it may be too late to fertilize the egg. This is why BBT charts are often difficult to use for ovulation prediction. Once the BBT rises the temperature should stay elevated until the onset of menstrual bleeding. If the woman becomes pregnant, the elevated temperature continues past the day of expected bleeding.

With the introduction of the ovulation-prediction kits, BBT charting has been replaced as the mainstay for ovulation prediction. However, there are a few remaining advantages of BBT charts: the cost and learning about your cycle. A BBT chart is cheap because it can be performed at the cost of a good thermometer and the paper used to make the graph. Most helpful is to use your BBT chart as a tool to measure the length of your cycle, to help establish if you are ovulating, and to find out approximately when in the previous month you ovulated. This information can help you decide what day to start testing with the ovulation-prediction kits in subsequent cycles. I have included a sample blank BBT chart at the end of this chapter for you to use. But you should always remember that the body is not a clock, and you may not ovulate on exactly the same day from cycle to cycle. Use the BBT chart as an excellent way to better understand your menstrual cycles, but I recommend using ovulation-prediction kits specifically for ovulation prediction. Therefore, BBT charts are not nearly as useful in predicting ovulation as they are in *looking back to see when you ovulated in previous months*.

If you do decide to use BBT charts to predict ovulation, don't be frustrated if you have trouble reading it. A study by Dr. Joan Bauman from the Masters & Johnson Institute asked six different expert physicians to separately review the BBT charts from 77 women who were ovulating. Using the BBT charts, this panel of experts was only able to accurately predict the day of ovulation (plus or minus one day) in 22.1 percent of the women. The temperature change in the other women was so subtle that even "expert" physicians were unable to pinpoint ovulation. *Compare the accuracy of the BBT charts— 22.1 percent even in the hands of experts—with the 90 percent predictive accuracy of the ovulation-prediction kits.*

The BBT chart requires a good quality thermometer that reads in tenths of a degree (for example, 98.2, 98.3). You must use the thermometer every day of the cycle, starting on the first day of your menstrual period (cycle day 1). You should take your temperature as soon as you wake up in the morning, before getting out of bed. *Do not even walk to another room*, such as the bathroom—this activity can raise your temperature enough to invalidate the chart. Remember that 98.6 degrees Fahrenheit (37 degrees Celsius) is the average body temperature of humans, but your average temperature may be a degree or more higher or lower and still be considered normal.

Figure 5.5A / A BBT Chart Consistent with Ovulation

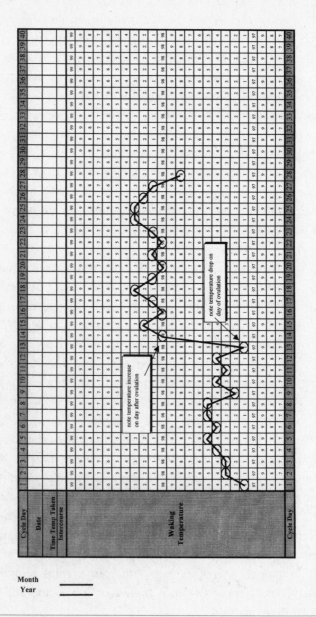

A BBT chart that shows two distinct plateaus or levels of temperature (lower in the first half of the cycle and higher in the second half) is referred to as biphasic and indicates that you probably did ovulate that month. The distinct temperature plateaus, as well as the drop in temperature before the rise, is indicated in Figure 5.5A. If the chart does not appear to be biphasic (Figure 5.5B) then *(continued)*

Figure 5.5B / A BBT Chart Consistent with No Ovulation

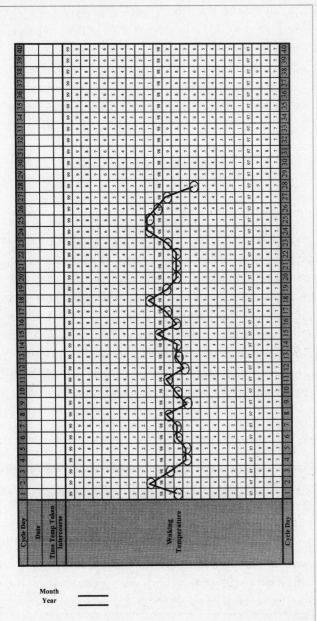

it suggests that you may not have ovulated that month. However, some women have more subtle alterations in their temperature and do ovulate despite BBT charts that are not biphasic. *The bottom line is that when BBT charts look like Figure 5.5A then that is good evidence that you ovulated that month, and looking back at the chart you should be able to estimate which day you ovulated.*

If you decide to use BBT charts, use them for one month and see if they work for you. You will likely not recognize the drop in temperature—the optimal time for intercourse—until the subsequent temperature rise occurs. However, this information can be applied to your next cycle to plan your intercourse and/or decide when to start using your ovulation-prediction kit. If you have trouble interpreting your charts, don't be frustrated. Don't use them for more than a few months—switch to another method of ovulation prediction instead.

When to Have Sex Using BBT Charts

My recommendations for frequency of sexual intercourse for couples using BBT charts are similar to those for couples using ovulation-prediction kits. Have intercourse every 36 to 48 hours until you recognize the subtle drop in temperature or the subsequent rise—whichever you note first. Then have intercourse every 24 hours beginning that day and continuing for two more days. If you do not recognize the temperature drop but note the temperature rise, it may already be too late to conceive, but you should have intercourse that day.

Using Basal-Body-Temperature Charts

- Use a good quality thermometer—one with tenths of a degree clearly marked. (Digital thermometers are probably the best.)
- Take your temperature *every day before you get out of bed*.
- *If you see a drop in the basal-body-temperature chart, have intercourse that day and the next day.* You should also have intercourse a third time, on the second day after the temperature drop, but it is not as crucial.

- If you miss the temperature drop, have intercourse on the first day you recognize the temperature rise and again the day after, 24 hours apart.
- Do not use BBT charts to achieve pregnancy for more than a few months (cycles).

CERVICAL MUCUS CHANGES

Occasionally patients ask me about the relationship between the changes in the thickness of their vaginal secretions and the timing of ovulation. The cervical mucus, which makes up the majority of the fluid from the vagina, is a fairly good marker of estrogen levels in the body and can help you know when you are in your most fertile period. As the estrogen level rises in the first half of your cycle, your mucus changes from a minimal amount of thick, sticky mucus, to a plentiful, thin, watery consistency that is slippery to the feel. Ovulation occurs when the copious, thin discharge is present.

To check your cervical mucus consistency, place your index and middle fingers into your vagina and feel at the end of the vagina for the round, firm cervix. Your cervix will feel about as firm as the end of your nose. In the center of the cervix is the cervical os (or opening of the cervical canal), which feels like a dimple. Collect the cervical mucus from the dimple in the middle of the cervix on the end of your finger. Note the appearance of the mucus—around the time of ovulation the mucus should be watery, slippery, and thin. Between your thumb and index or middle finger, stretch the mucus. You should be able to pull it apart at least three inches (eight centimeters) during your most fertile time.

There are some reasons why testing cervical mucus is not

the optimal method for predicting ovulation in most women. One is that the rise in estrogen levels can last for up to one week, and therefore the changes in a woman's cervical mucus produced by this rise only roughly approximates her day of ovulation. Additionally, these mucus changes are quite subjective and there is a substantial amount of variation among women. Finally, testing cervical mucus is a messy method that some women may prefer to forgo in favor of other methods. The use of cervical mucus changes has been promoted by many books, because it is a more "natural" method of prediction and because BBT charts used to be the only other option and had many limitations of their own.

I know of no study, similar to the one by Dr. Bauman noted earlier, where a panel of physician experts tried to predict ovulation by evaluating cervical mucus changes in a group of women. I assume that if a study was completed it would have results poorer than the 22.1 percent accuracy estimated for BBT charts. However, for many women cervical mucus changes can be useful to know when to start having intercourse every other day in anticipation of ovulation.

"MITTELSCHMERZ"

Some women are able to recognize the day each month when ovulation occurs. On this day, they feel pain on the side of their pelvis where ovulation is occurring. This mid-cycle pain associated with ovulation is referred to as *"mittelschmerz."* *Mittelschmerz* is a German term that means "middle pain." Ovulation occurs from only one ovary each month, but it is random which side it will be. Just because ovulation occurred on one side does not mean that the next month ovulation will occur on the opposite side. It's just like flipping a coin, where two or three heads in a row would not be unexpected.

It is estimated that up to 25 percent of women experience *mittelschmerz* at least intermittently. If you are a woman who experiences regular, predictable monthly pain, you may be able to use this as an indicator to time your intercourse. Because there are many other abdominal pains that can be confused with *mittelschmerz*, I suggest that you correlate the discomfort associated with your ovulation with another mode of ovulation prediction, such as the over-the-counter kits or BBT charts. This will confirm that you are, in fact, experiencing *mittelschmerz*. Since this discomfort is regularly noted by only a small percentage of women, this method will not be reliable.

OTHER AVAILABLE TECHNOLOGIES

Two other technologies have been mass-marketed to assist couples with ovulation prediction: the Clearblue Easy Fertility Monitor, and the CUE ovulation predictor. These methods use novel techniques to predict ovulation, and both can be used at home.

The Clearblue Easy Fertility Monitor is a machine the size of an electronic planner that interprets daily urine samples. The monitor tells you which days to supply urine samples for testing each cycle. You simply hold a disposable testing stick in your urine stream, then place the stick in the monitor. The monitor measures both estrogen levels and luteinizing hormone (LH) levels to predict ovulation. On the screen of the monitor your "fertility status" is displayed, indicating when ovulation will occur. Presumably, the combination of LH and estrogen measurements makes this the most accurate at-home way to predict ovulation. The Clearblue Easy Fertility Monitor is expensive, retailing at about $200, plus $50 for the test sticks. Since the basic ovulation-prediction kits are only around $30 and, when used properly, are around 90 percent accurate (greater than 95 percent accurate if used twice a day), it is difficult to justify the expense involved in the purchase of one of these new monitors. However, if you suspect that it may take more than six months to become pregnant, you have very irregular cycles (more than 35 days but less than 42 days in length, according to the manufacturer), or you have previously had problems using the ovulation-predictor kits, then this monitor may be the right method for you.

One of the pediatricians I work with asked me what the best way is to time your intercourse appropriately with ovulation. I asked her if cost was a consideration, and she replied, "Not really." My answer to her was that if you have money to spend and want the Cadillac of ovulation prediction, then the Clearblue Easy Fertility Monitor is probably what you are looking for. More information can be obtained by visiting their website, *www.clearblueeasy.com*, or by calling 1 (800) 321–EASY.

The CUE ovulation predictor uses salivary and cervical mucus samples to evaluate electrolyte and electrical resistance changes that coincide with ovulation. It requires placing a test sensor in your mouth to obtain a sample of saliva and inserting a probe into the vagina to obtain a sample of cervical mucus. The electronic monitor calculates and charts oral and vaginal electrical resistance measurements (in the saliva and cervical mucus). The woman provides salivary samples every day, whereas she starts the vaginal samples on cycle day 8 and continues until ovulation. Changes in the electrical resistance of these body fluids have been shown to be reliably predictive of ovulation.

Apparently the CUE method predicts ovulation about five to seven days in advance by the oral salivary samples and uses the vaginal mucus samples to indicate the precise day of ovulation. There are no studies I am aware of that compare the CUE to the ovulation-prediction kits, so it is uncertain how they compare. The CUE is rarely used by my patients because it is more invasive and complicated than the other methods and is also the most expensive method at about $495. However, CUE can also be rented at $45 monthly plus shipping and handling and a refundable deposit. More information can be obtained by calling 1 (800) 367-2837 or visiting their website, *www.zetek-inc.com*. Other ovulation-tracking devices include the OV Watch and OvaCue Fertility Monitor. The OV Watch has a sensor that measures the amount of chloride a woman produces in her sweat. The watch is worn at night while sleeping. The watch and sensors cost about $250 and can be found at *www.ovwatch.com*. The OvaCue Fertility Monitor is an electronic device that measures the changes in the electrolytes found in saliva to predict ovulation. This device costs close to $300.

My recommendation is that if you are trying to determine when an LH surge is occurring then use the products that measure LH directly. Using sweat, saliva, temperature, or cervical mucus changes to indirectly determine the LH rise, and timing of ovulation, may be less accurate.

LUTEAL PHASE DEFICIENCY (LPD)

One concept that I want to introduce is called luteal phase deficiency. As we reviewed in this chapter, the luteal phase is the second part of the menstrual cycle and begins after the rise in LH and ends with the onset of menstrual bleeding. This part of the menstrual cycle is a vitally important period that is fairly fixed in duration, lasting 14 days, plus or minus two days. A short luteal phase is one that lasts less than 12 days and is referred to as luteal phase deficiency. Because a normal luteal phase is vital for implantation and early growth of the embryo, LPD increases the risk of infertility and miscarriage. After applying some of the methods reviewed above to establish the day of your ovulation and the length of your menstrual cycles you may identify a short luteal phase. Because LPD is very commonly seen in athletic and thin women, it is discussed in detail in Chapter 6.

Figure 5.6

OVULATION PREDICTION METHODS

METHOD	RELIABILITY	PROS	CONS	RECOMMENDATIONS
Ovulation-prediction kit	very high (about 90% accuracy when used once daily; 95% when used twice daily)	• very accurate • fast • easy to perform • cost-effective	• $20–$40 per month • can sometimes be difficult to interpret	Most cost-effective ovulation prediction method—*probably the best for most women.*
BBT chart (basal body temperature)	poor as a prospective tool	inexpensive (the cost of a good thermometer)	• inaccurate • requires daily measurements • can be frustrating to interpret	Useful to determine cycle length, and at the end of a cycle to determine whether ovulation took place. May be helpful in preparation for using ovulation-prediction kit.
Cervical mucus	poor	no cost	• only indicates ovulation to within one week • highly subjective	Consider combining with a BBT chart to make both methods more accurate.
Recognizing mid-cycle pain ("*mittelschmerz*")	overall poor, however in a minority of women can be accurate	no cost	• pain may arise from other sources • most women cannot recognize this reliably	Should not rely on this method alone. If you want to use this method, confirm the pain with another more reliable method.
Clearblue Easy Fertility Monitor	very high	probably the most accurate method	$200–$250	If money is not an issue this is probably the best method.
CUE	very high	• very accurate • can be rented monthly	• $450 • more complicated to use than other methods • invasive	Consider monthly rental before purchasing.

Figure 5.7

BASAL-BODY-TEMPERATURE CHART

MONTH ____________

YEAR ____________

Cycle Day	1	2	3	4	5	6	7	8	9	10	11	12	13	14	15	16	17	18	19	20	21	22	23	24	25	26	27	28	29	30	31	32	33	34	35	36	37	38	39	40
Date																																								
Time Temp. Taken																																								
Intercourse																																								
	5	5	5	5	5	5	5	5	5	5	5	5	5	5	5	5	5	5	5	5	5	5	5	5	5	5	5	5	5	5	5	5	5	5	5	5	5	5	5	5
	4	4	4	4	4	4	4	4	4	4	4	4	4	4	4	4	4	4	4	4	4	4	4	4	4	4	4	4	4	4	4	4	4	4	4	4	4	4	4	4
	3	3	3	3	3	3	3	3	3	3	3	3	3	3	3	3	3	3	3	3	3	3	3	3	3	3	3	3	3	3	3	3	3	3	3	3	3	3	3	3
	2	2	2	2	2	2	2	2	2	2	2	2	2	2	2	2	2	2	2	2	2	2	2	2	2	2	2	2	2	2	2	2	2	2	2	2	2	2	2	2
	1	1	1	1	1	1	1	1	1	1	1	1	1	1	1	1	1	1	1	1	1	1	1	1	1	1	1	1	1	1	1	1	1	1	1	1	1	1	1	1
	99	99	99	99	99	99	99	99	99	99	99	99	99	99	99	99	99	99	99	99	99	99	99	99	99	99	99	99	99	99	99	99	99	99	99	99	99	99	99	99
	9	9	9	9	9	9	9	9	9	9	9	9	9	9	9	9	9	9	9	9	9	9	9	9	9	9	9	9	9	9	9	9	9	9	9	9	9	9	9	9
	8	8	8	8	8	8	8	8	8	8	8	8	8	8	8	8	8	8	8	8	8	8	8	8	8	8	8	8	8	8	8	8	8	8	8	8	8	8	8	8
	7	7	7	7	7	7	7	7	7	7	7	7	7	7	7	7	7	7	7	7	7	7	7	7	7	7	7	7	7	7	7	7	7	7	7	7	7	7	7	7
	6	6	6	6	6	6	6	6	6	6	6	6	6	6	6	6	6	6	6	6	6	6	6	6	6	6	6	6	6	6	6	6	6	6	6	6	6	6	6	6
	5	5	5	5	5	5	5	5	5	5	5	5	5	5	5	5	5	5	5	5	5	5	5	5	5	5	5	5	5	5	5	5	5	5	5	5	5	5	5	5
	4	4	4	4	4	4	4	4	4	4	4	4	4	4	4	4	4	4	4	4	4	4	4	4	4	4	4	4	4	4	4	4	4	4	4	4	4	4	4	4
Waking Temperature	3	3	3	3	3	3	3	3	3	3	3	3	3	3	3	3	3	3	3	3	3	3	3	3	3	3	3	3	3	3	3	3	3	3	3	3	3	3	3	3
	2	2	2	2	2	2	2	2	2	2	2	2	2	2	2	2	2	2	2	2	2	2	2	2	2	2	2	2	2	2	2	2	2	2	2	2	2	2	2	2
	1	1	1	1	1	1	1	1	1	1	1	1	1	1	1	1	1	1	1	1	1	1	1	1	1	1	1	1	1	1	1	1	1	1	1	1	1	1	1	1
	98	98	98	98	98	98	98	98	98	98	98	98	98	98	98	98	98	98	98	98	98	98	98	98	98	98	98	98	98	98	98	98	98	98	98	98	98	98	98	98
	9	9	9	9	9	9	9	9	9	9	9	9	9	9	9	9	9	9	9	9	9	9	9	9	9	9	9	9	9	9	9	9	9	9	9	9	9	9	9	9
	8	8	8	8	8	8	8	8	8	8	8	8	8	8	8	8	8	8	8	8	8	8	8	8	8	8	8	8	8	8	8	8	8	8	8	8	8	8	8	8
	7	7	7	7	7	7	7	7	7	7	7	7	7	7	7	7	7	7	7	7	7	7	7	7	7	7	7	7	7	7	7	7	7	7	7	7	7	7	7	7
	6	6	6	6	6	6	6	6	6	6	6	6	6	6	6	6	6	6	6	6	6	6	6	6	6	6	6	6	6	6	6	6	6	6	6	6	6	6	6	6
	5	5	5	5	5	5	5	5	5	5	5	5	5	5	5	5	5	5	5	5	5	5	5	5	5	5	5	5	5	5	5	5	5	5	5	5	5	5	5	5
	4	4	4	4	4	4	4	4	4	4	4	4	4	4	4	4	4	4	4	4	4	4	4	4	4	4	4	4	4	4	4	4	4	4	4	4	4	4	4	4
	3	3	3	3	3	3	3	3	3	3	3	3	3	3	3	3	3	3	3	3	3	3	3	3	3	3	3	3	3	3	3	3	3	3	3	3	3	3	3	3
	2	2	2	2	2	2	2	2	2	2	2	2	2	2	2	2	2	2	2	2	2	2	2	2	2	2	2	2	2	2	2	2	2	2	2	2	2	2	2	2
	1	1	1	1	1	1	1	1	1	1	1	1	1	1	1	1	1	1	1	1	1	1	1	1	1	1	1	1	1	1	1	1	1	1	1	1	1	1	1	1
	97	97	97	97	97	97	97	97	97	97	97	97	97	97	97	97	97	97	97	97	97	97	97	97	97	97	97	97	97	97	97	97	97	97	97	97	97	97	97	97
	9	9	9	9	9	9	9	9	9	9	9	9	9	9	9	9	9	9	9	9	9	9	9	9	9	9	9	9	9	9	9	9	9	9	9	9	9	9	9	9
	8	8	8	8	8	8	8	8	8	8	8	8	8	8	8	8	8	8	8	8	8	8	8	8	8	8	8	8	8	8	8	8	8	8	8	8	8	8	8	8
	7	7	7	7	7	7	7	7	7	7	7	7	7	7	7	7	7	7	7	7	7	7	7	7	7	7	7	7	7	7	7	7	7	7	7	7	7	7	7	7
	6	6	6	6	6	6	6	6	6	6	6	6	6	6	6	6	6	6	6	6	6	6	6	6	6	6	6	6	6	6	6	6	6	6	6	6	6	6	6	6
	5	5	5	5	5	5	5	5	5	5	5	5	5	5	5	5	5	5	5	5	5	5	5	5	5	5	5	5	5	5	5	5	5	5	5	5	5	5	5	5
Cycle Day	1	2	3	4	5	6	7	8	9	10	11	12	13	14	15	16	17	18	19	20	21	22	23	24	25	26	27	28	29	30	31	32	33	34	35	36	37	38	39	40

6

Weight and Exercise

IT'S no secret that the majority of Americans are outside the accepted ranges for their weight. Just stop and look around the next time you go to the grocery store or the mall. Some of us are too thin, but more than half of us are overweight. What many people don't realize is that being overweight or underweight has a profound influence on a woman's fertility and may also affect pregnancy outcome.

Exercise can also be a source of fertility problems. Moderate regular exercise is healthy and fertility enhancing, but excessive exercise, along with the reduced body fat and body weight it may cause, can dramatically decrease fertility and can also increase miscarriage rates. I have chosen to discuss exercise and weight in the same chapter because these two concerns are closely related. This chapter addresses these fertility issues only in the female partner; weight and exercise, unless at severe extremes (such as starvation), have little effect on male fertility.

ARE YOU OUTSIDE THE ACCEPTED
WEIGHT RANGE FOR YOUR HEIGHT?

An American woman is more likely than not to be outside the normal expected weight range for her height. More than 50 percent of American women are overweight for their height, and about 10 percent of American women are considered underweight. This means that more than half of all American women need to alter their weight to maximize their health.

To begin with, each reader needs to decide whether her own weight falls outside the normal range. In Figure 6.1, you can plot your height and weight to determine your body mass index (BMI). The BMI is a very easy and accurate tool to discover whether you are overweight or underweight. If you want to determine your BMI more precisely you can use the following formula, but I think the graph is easier. BMI = (your weight in pounds divided by 2.2) divided by (your height in inches times $0.0254)^2$ or, in metric units: BMI = (your weight in kilograms) divided by (your height in meters)^2. The resulting BMI indicates:

- You are underweight if your BMI is less than 20;
- You have a normal weight for your height if your BMI is between 20 and 24.9;
- You are overweight if your BMI is greater than or equal to 25 (some sources say 26);
- You are considered obese if your BMI is greater than or equal to 30 (some sources say 29).

Next, I would like every reader to take a few minutes to determine their body-fat percentage. A simple yet surprisingly accurate method (plus or minus 2 to 4 percent) of determining your body fat can be done at home with nothing more than a measuring tape. Using a measuring tape you need to measure

Figure 6.1

BODY-MASS INDEX CHART

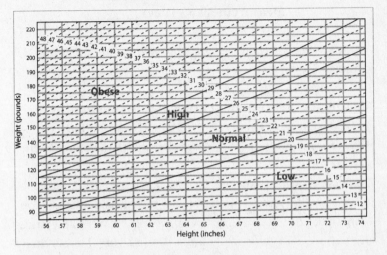

With permission from the Institute of Medicine. Subcommittee for a Clinical Application Guide, Committee on Nutritional Status During Pregnancy and Lactation, Food and Nutrition Board, and the National Academy of Sciences. "Nutrition during pregnancy and lactation." Washington, D.C.: National Academy Press. Copyright © 1992.

three parts of your body and then write the numbers in the blanks below. The measurements are then used in a simple formula to give you a special number called a Measurement Conversion Number. This number is then plugged into Figure 6.2 and you will have your estimated body-fat percentage. It's not hard at all to do, just follow the directions below.

Measurement #1: Measure the circumference of your abdomen at the thinnest part of your waist.

Measurement #1 (waist)_____

Measurement #2: Measure the circumference of your hips at the level of the widest protrusion of your buttocks.

Measurement #2 (hips)_____

Measurement #3: Measure the circumference of your neck—just below the level of the voice box (Adam's apple)

Measurement #3 (neck)_____

Once you have the three measurements, plug them into the formula below.

Finding the Measurement Conversion Number:

Measurement #1 (waist)_____ + Measurement #2 (hips)_____ −
Measurement #3 (neck)_____ = Measurement Conversion Number

Double-check to make sure you subtracted the neck measurement from the sum of the waist and hip measurements. Now, simply take the Measurement Conversion Number you calculated above and refer to Figure 6.2. Find your Measurement Conversion Number in the appropriate row in the far left column. Then look across the row until you intersect with the column containing your height (found on the top row). The corresponding number is your estimated body-fat percentage. It's as simple as that.

OVERWEIGHT

Developed nations such as the U.S. have noted a staggering increase in obesity during the second half of the twentieth century. The availability of high-calorie foods at reasonable prices, combined with a sedentary lifestyle, has led to an epidemic of obesity. This trend has dramatically worsened over the last 30 years in the U.S. with at least 10 percent more women now in the overweight category than in the 1970s. This is despite an estimated $30 billion spent annually on the diet industry, a federally sponsored health program to reduce

Figure 6.2
BODY-FAT PERCENTAGE ESTIMATION FOR WOMEN

Measurement Conversion Number*

	60.5	61	61.5	62	62.5	63	63.5	64	64.5	65	65.5	66	66.5	67	67.5	68	68.5	69	69.5	70	70.5	71	71.5	72
36.5	3	2	2	2	1	1	1	0																
37	4	3	3	3	2	2	2	1	1	0														
37.5	5	4	4	4	3	3	3	2	2	2	1	1	1	0										
38	6	5	5	5	4	4	3	3	3	2	2	2	1	1	0									
38.5	7	6	6	5	5	5	4	4	4	3	3	3	2	2	2	1	1	1	0	0				
39	7	7	7	6	6	6	5	5	5	4	4	4	3	3	3	2	2	2	1	1	1	0	0	
39.5	8	8	8	7	7	7	6	6	6	5	5	5	4	4	4	3	3	3	2	2	2	1	1	
40	9	9	8	8	8	7	7	7	6	6	6	5	5	5	4	4	4	3	3	3	3	2	2	
40.5	10	10	9	9	9	8	8	8	7	7	7	6	6	6	5	5	5	4	4	4	3	3	3	2
41	11	11	10	10	10	9	9	8	8	8	7	7	7	6	6	6	5	5	5	4	4	4	3	
41.5	12	11	11	11	10	10	10	9	9	9	8	8	8	7	7	7	6	6	6	5	5	5	4	4
42	13	12	12	12	11	11	10	10	10	9	9	9	8	8	8	7	7	7	6	6	6	5	5	
42.5	13	13	13	12	12	12	11	11	11	10	10	10	9	9	9	8	8	8	7	7	7	6	6	6
43	14	14	14	13	13	12	12	12	11	11	11	10	10	10	9	9	9	8	8	8	7	7	7	
43.5	15	15	14	14	14	13	13	13	12	12	12	11	11	11	10	10	10	9	9	9	8	8	8	7
44	16	16	15	15	14	14	13	13	13	12	12	12	11	11	10	10	10	9	9	9	8	8		
44.5	17	16	16	16	15	15	15	14	14	14	13	13	13	12	12	12	11	11	11	11	10	10	10	9
45	17	17	17	16	16	15	15	15	14	14	14	13	13	13	12	12	12	11	11	11	11	10	10	10
45.5	18	18	18	17	17	16	16	16	15	15	15	14	14	14	13	13	13	12	12	12	12	11	11	11
46	19	19	18	18	18	17	17	17	16	16	16	15	15	15	14	14	14	13	13	13	13	12	12	11
46.5	20	19	19	19	18	18	18	17	17	17	16	16	16	15	15	15	14	14	14	13	13	13	13	12
47	20	20	20	19	19	19	18	18	18	17	17	17	16	16	16	15	15	15	14	14	14	13	13	13
47.5	21	21	21	20	20	19	19	19	18	18	18	17	17	17	16	16	16	15	15	15	15	14	14	14
48	22	22	21	21	21	20	20	20	19	19	19	18	18	18	17	17	17	16	16	16	16	15	15	15
48.5	23	22	22	22	21	21	21	20	20	20	19	19	19	18	18	18	17	17	17	16	16	16	15	15
49	23	23	23	22	22	22	21	21	21	20	20	20	19	19	19	18	18	18	17	17	17	16	16	16
49.5	24	24	24	23	23	22	22	22	21	21	21	20	20	20	19	19	19	18	18	18	17	17	17	17
50	25	24	24	24	23	23	23	22	22	22	21	21	21	20	20	20	19	19	19	18	18	18	18	
50.5	26	25	25	25	24	24	23	23	23	23	22	22	22	21	21	21	20	20	20	19	19	19	19	
51	26	26	26	25	25	25	24	24	24	23	23	23	22	22	22	21	21	21	20	20	20	19	19	19
51.5	27	27	26	26	26	25	25	25	24	24	24	23	23	23	22	22	22	21	21	21	20	20	20	20
52	28	27	27	27	26	26	26	25	25	25	24	24	24	23	23	23	22	22	22	21	21	21	21	20
52.5	28	28	28	27	27	27	26	26	26	25	25	25	24	24	24	23	23	23	22	22	22	22	21	21
53	29	29	28	28	28	27	27	27	26	26	26	25	25	25	25	24	24	24	23	23	23	22	22	22
53.5	30	29	29	29	28	28	28	27	27	27	26	26	26	25	25	25	25	24	24	24	23	23	23	22
54	30	30	30	29	29	29	28	28	28	27	27	27	26	26	26	25	25	25	25	24	24	24	24	
54.5	31	31	30	30	30	29	29	29	28	28	28	27	27	27	26	26	26	25	25	25	25	24	24	24
55	32	31	31	31	30	30	30	29	29	29	28	28	28	27	27	27	26	26	26	25	25	25	25	
55.5	32	32	32	31	31	31	30	30	30	29	29	29	28	28	28	27	27	27	26	26	26	25	25	25
56	33	33	32	32	32	31	31	31	30	30	30	30	29	29	29	28	28	28	27	27	27	26	26	26
56.5	34	33	33	33	32	32	32	31	31	31	30	30	30	29	29	29	29	28	28	28	27	27	27	26
57	34	34	34	33	33	32	32	32	31	31	31	30	30	30	29	29	29	29	28	28	28	27	27	27
57.5	35	34	34	34	33	33	33	32	32	32	31	31	31	30	30	30	29	29	29	29	28	28	28	27
58	35	35	35	34	34	34	33	33	33	32	32	32	31	31	31	31	30	30	30	29	29	29	29	
58.5	36	36	35	35	35	34	34	34	33	33	33	32	32	32	31	31	31	31	30	30	30	29	29	29
59	37	36	36	36	35	35	35	34	34	34	33	33	33	32	32	32	32	31	31	31	30	30	30	29
59.5	37	37	37	36	36	35	35	35	34	34	34	33	33	33	33	32	32	32	31	31	31	30	30	30
60	38	37	37	37	36	36	36	35	35	35	34	34	34	34	33	33	33	32	32	32	32	31	31	30
60.5	38	38	38	37	37	37	36	36	36	35	35	35	34	34	34	33	33	33	33	32	32	32	31	31
61	39	39	38	38	38	37	37	37	36	36	36	35	35	35	34	34	34	34	33	33	33	32	32	32
61.5	40	39	39	39	38	38	38	37	37	37	36	36	36	35	35	35	35	34	34	34	33	33	33	32
62	40	40	39	39	39	38	38	38	37	37	37	36	36	36	36	35	35	35	34	34	34	34	33	33
62.5	41	40	40	40	39	39	39	38	38	38	37	37	37	36	36	36	36	35	35	35	34	34	34	34
63	41	41	41	40	40	40	39	39	39	38	38	38	37	37	37	37	36	36	36	35	35	35	35	34
63.5	42	41	41	41	40	40	40	40	39	39	39	38	38	38	37	37	37	37	36	36	36	35	35	35
64	42	42	42	41	41	41	40	40	40	39	39	39	38	38	38	38	37	37	37	36	36	36	36	35
64.5	43	43	42	42	42	41	41	41	40	40	40	39	39	39	38	38	38	38	37	37	37	36	36	36
65	43	43	43	42	42	42	41	41	41	40	40	40	39	39	39	39	38	38	38	37	37	37	36	36
65.5	44	44	43	43	43	42	42	42	41	41	41	41	40	40	40	39	39	39	38	38	38	37	37	37
66	45	44	44	44	43	43	43	42	42	42	41	41	41	41	40	40	40	39	39	39	38	38	38	37
66.5	45	45	44	44	44	43	43	43	42	42	42	41	41	41	41	40	40	40	39	39	39	38	38	38
67	46	45	45	45	44	44	44	43	43	43	42	42	42	42	41	41	41	40	40	40	39	39	39	38
67.5	46	46	45	45	45	44	44	44	43	43	43	43	42	42	42	41	41	41	41	40	40	40	39	39
68	47	46	46	46	45	45	45	44	44	44	43	43	43	42	42	42	41	41	41	41	40	40	40	39
68.5		47	46	46	46	45	45	45	44	44	44	43	43	43	42	42	42	41	41	41	41	40	40	40
69			47	47	46	46	46	45	45	45	44	44	44	43	43	43	42	42	42	41	41	41	41	40
69.5				47	46	46	46	45	45	45	44	44	44	43	43	43	43	42	42	42	41	41	41	41
70					47	47	46	46	46	45	45	45	44	44	44	44	43	43	43	43	42	42	42	41

* Measurement Conversion Number=waist+hip-neck circumference (in inches)

With permission from the Naval Health Research Center, San Diego, Calif. J. A. Hogdgon and M. B. Beckett. "Prediction of Percent Body Fat for U.S. Navy Women from Body Circumferences and Height." *NHRC Report* no. 84-29 the prevalence of overweight by the year 2000, and the so-called fitness craze that began in the 1970s.

Being overweight is a common and indisputable cause of irregular periods and reduced fertility. Dr. Robert Norman, an Australian expert on weight and fertility, commented during a lecture at the 1999 American Society of Reproductive Medicine National Meeting that in his infertile population about 60 percent of the women are significantly overweight. This is substantially higher than the normal percentage for a group of women in their reproductive years. Even being modestly overweight, with a BMI of 25 to 29, reduces your chances of getting pregnant within a reasonable amount of time by about one-third. A study in 1998 by Dr. Francine Grodstein and colleagues at Harvard University School of Public Health determined that *women with a BMI of greater than or equal to 27 were over three times more likely than women of normal weight to have infertility caused by problems with ovulation.*

Overweight women frequently have difficulty believing that their weight could be reducing their fertility. For example, I recently heard the following comment from an obese patient with irregular cycles: "I don't think my weight has anything to do with it. My friend weighs twenty-five pounds more than I do and she's had two kids."

Hormonal Changes with Weight Gain

The causes of obesity-related infertility are still poorly understood, but we do know that many overweight women develop hormonal irregularities that trigger irregular or absent menstrual cycles. Polycystic ovarian syndrome (PCOS) (discussed in detail in Chapter 2) is a good example of a common fertility problem often triggered by weight gain.

Some women are very sensitive to excess body fat, so gaining even a moderate amount of weight may result in problems with their reproductive system. The brain recognizes the amount of fat in the body by the levels of hormones such as leptin and insulin circulating in the bloodstream. These hormone levels rise as the amount of body fat increases. In some genetically predisposed women, levels of these hormones increase out of proportion to weight gain. The problem is that abnormal levels of leptin and insulin in the bloodstream directly, and indirectly, affect the function of the ovaries and therefore are believed to exert a significant influence on fertility.

Other women don't have the genetic predisposition for these hormonal changes with weight gain, so their increased weight may not significantly alter their hormones or menstrual cycles. If menstrual cycles stay very regular and predictable despite weight

Figure 6.3

THE RELATIONSHIP BETWEEN WEIGHT AND FERTILITY

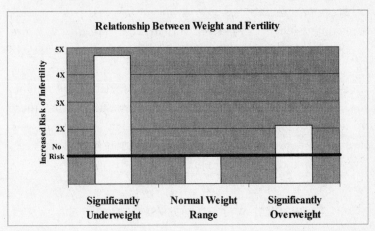

B. B. Green, N. S. Weiss, and J. R. Daling. "Risk of Ovulatory Infertility in Relation to Body Weight." *Fertility and Sterility* 50 (1988): 721–26. Copyright © 1988, Elsevier Science.

gain, a woman's fertility has probably not been affected. But you should remember that *obesity is associated with miscarriage* (reviewed below) *and many serious pregnancy complications— such as diabetes, hypertension, and cesarean section—that can result in high-risk pregnancies and possibly lifelong problems for both the mother and the baby.* In a perfect world, all obstetricians would like to have their patients be in the normal weight range before they become pregnant. I realize this can be a daunting task, but even a modest weight loss of 5 percent of your total body weight has been shown to be worthwhile.

A Link Between Miscarriage and Overweight?

Being overweight may also be a significant risk factor for miscarriage. In 1998, Dr. A. M. Clark and colleagues from the University of Adelaide in Australia published a study that suggested an important connection between obesity and miscarriage. They provided 67 obese women with intense diet and exercise therapy for six months prior to becoming pregnant. *In previous pregnancies, before the weight-loss intervention, the women had a 75 percent miscarriage rate; this loss rate dropped to 18 percent after their weight reduction.* Studies of women with PCOS (most women with this problem are significantly overweight) have also shown an association with higher risk of miscarriage. It is important to say studies like these do not prove causation. Further research will need to be performed to better understand this association between excessive weight and miscarriage and the underlying causes.

GENERAL WEIGHT-LOSS SUGGESTIONS

Now that I have convinced you that excessive weight can undermine fertility in many women, what can be done about it?

If I had the answer to that question for all women, this would be a best-selling diet book instead of a fertility book. However, there are some basic rules that all effective weight-loss plans share, and we will go over these together. In addition, women with PCOS often find that a specific category of diet, the low-carbohydrate, high-protein diet, is particularly valuable for them. A modified American Diabetes Association diet is probably an excellent choice. This specific diet has been shown to be an effective means of weight loss in a general population, but I want to highlight its role in women with PCOS.

Successful weight loss involves much more than just changing your diet. In this chapter, I will review the other vital components of a successful weight loss program. Remember, if you decide to start dieting, it is always recommended that you visit your physician first for an evaluation.

Which Diet Is Best?

Most diet books claim that their novel approach takes advantage of a unique aspect of metabolism, digestion, motivation, or physiology to make it more successful than other diets. For an individual, some strategies may be more effective than others, but regardless of which one you choose, the unifying theme of dieting is very straightforward: if you burn more calories than you consume, you will lose weight. Whether you are on a protein diet, rice diet, liquid diet, low-fat diet, Weight Watchers, or any other diet, they all work when the calories consumed are fewer than the calories expended. This means you can either restrict the calories that you take in or increase your activity so that you're burning more calories than you eat. Of course, the best strategy is to combine exercise with calorie restriction.

In my experience most people recognize the importance of caloric restriction and exercise for successful weight loss, but the majority of dieters are looking for an easier way out. The testimonials from those who have tried fad diets and have lost substantial amounts of weight with apparent ease are so much more compelling and interesting. If you pay attention to the diet fads over the years you will notice that the same ones come and go, resurrected every ten or fifteen years.

There are no magical foods or combinations that offer the optimal diet strategy for everyone. Many people believe that the carbohydrate or fat content of the food they consume is what determines whether they will gain weight. In 1992, a study by Dr. Rudolph Leibel, Dr. Jules Hirsch, and colleagues at the Centers for Disease Control (CDC) was published in the *American Journal of Clinical Nutrition*. The subjects were put on a special ward where every calorie was monitored. The fat content of their food was varied from 0 percent to 70 percent. The only factor that influenced their weight gain or loss was the total number of calories consumed; the fat content made no difference. In reality, a diet of cake and ice cream would be effective in weight loss if the total number of calories consumed was less than that required by the body.

Although the general philosophy of low-calorie dieting is most important (consuming fewer calories than your body uses), it is an oversimplified view. Different foods elicit distinct metabolic responses in the body. Combinations of foods and the ratio of food groups consumed appear to be important considerations in effective weight loss also. Because everyone has a unique physiology, specific diets may work better in some individuals than in others. Certainly, personal food preferences may be key to the success of a diet. Motivation is also a vital factor that is used successfully by many diets. For these and many other reasons a different best-selling diet book seems to come out every month.

How do you know which diet to choose? Let's examine the

"low-fat" diet fad that just ended. Americans have learned the hard way that "fat-free" or "low-fat" doesn't mean "no weight gain." Most low-fat foods are high carbohydrate sources, and excess carbohydrates consumed in the diet are converted to fat in the body. In this way, many "low-fat" dieters were breaking the first rule of dieting—they were eating more calories than they burned, so they gained weight. In the same study from the CDC noted earlier, 40 percent of low-fat dieters did not reduce their calories while restricting their fat intake. This is not to say that a "low-fat" diet can't work, *but if you do choose a low-fat diet then it must also be a low-calorie diet.*

The latest rage is a high-protein, low-carbohydrate diet. The books that promote this strategy assert that carbohydrates are the key to being overweight. On the other hand, vegetarians eat a very high-carbohydrate, low-protein diet, and I have yet to meet an obese vegetarian. So from this example and the others above, you can see that many seemingly diverse diets can be effective. This just reinforces the fact that no matter which diet you choose, you should always keep calories in mind and pick a diet you think you can stick to for the long haul.

Selecting a diet that meshes well with your own tastes and preferences is vital if you are going to stay with it. Some women need the structure of a Weight Watchers or Jenny Craig program, a registered dietitian, or close follow-up by a physician in order to be successful. Others may have trouble restricting their food intake and will want to try a diet like Dr. Atkins's high-protein diet, where your amounts of food are not restricted. Some women do not want to give up many of their favorite foods, and so a diet with reduced portion sizes of their normal meals might be the best choice. There is no one right diet for everyone, so individualize the choice until it is a good fit for you.

Dieting for Women with PCOS

One group of patients for whom I do recommend a specific diet is overweight women with PCOS. This condition is the most common hormonal problem of reproductive-age women and the most common fertility problem associated with being overweight. Experts have estimated that at least 5 percent of reproductive-age women have PCOS (at least one in 20 young women you pass on the street). Polycystic ovarian syndrome has also been associated with the possibility of a higher risk of miscarriage. In my clinic not a day goes by that I don't see a woman with PCOS.

I discussed PCOS in detail in Chapter 2; here I will focus on the dietary needs of women with PCOS, with an emphasis on effective weight-loss strategies. Combining these dietary recommendations with regular exercise is the first line of therapy for PCOS and will often correct the problem.

If you are overweight and have irregular menstrual periods and the other common symptoms of PCOS (unwanted or excessive hair growth and/or acne), weight loss will probably be your most effective treatment. The good news is that *in the case of PCOS, a modest weight loss (5 percent of your present weight) may be all you need to significantly improve your fertility.* The metabolic changes that occur when you alter your diet, shed a few pounds, and begin an exercise program can end PCOS. On the other hand, if you have symptoms of PCOS and your menstrual periods have been absent for more than three months, your bleeding is too frequent or very heavy, or you simply want to confirm the condition, I recommend you see your physician first, *before* attempting weight-loss therapy.

I routinely send all my PCOS patients to a registered dietician for an evaluation and counseling. A visit to a local registered dietitian is worthwhile to discuss an appropriate diet for someone with PCOS. Call ahead first to make sure the dietitian is familiar with PCOS and insulin resistance.

In my experience, the best diet for PCOS is whatever diet a woman can continue for the long term. Whether it is Weight Watchers, South Beach, or just restricting portion sizes, almost any diet can work. If you don't know what to do with your diet, then some version of a high-protein, low-carbohydrate diet, or a diabetic-type diet, is my suggestion. The dietary recommendations from the American Diabetes Association would be an excellent choice. In the general population these diets appear to be effective at promoting weight loss, but they are particularly appropriate for women with PCOS due to their insulin-lowering effects. One word of caution, though, is that the high-protein, low-carbohydrate diets seem to be successful for the short term but may not allow a reasonable dietary lifestyle for most people to continue it long term. The more restrictive the diet the less likely you will be able to continue it.

How Do Low-Carbohydrate, High-Protein Diets Work?

In order to learn about the low-carbohydrate, high-protein diets, first we need a basic understanding of how food is metabolized. There are three classes of food: proteins, carbohydrates, and fats. Carbohydrates make up about 70 percent of the normal American diet; they are the main source of energy used by the body. Excess carbohydrates become fat. When an inadequate number of calories are consumed in the diet, the body begins to break down fat stores for its energy. This is when permanent weight loss occurs. What are carbohydrates? One of my patients summed it up fairly well by saying, "If it tastes good it probably has a lot of 'carbs' in it." Basically, carbohydrates include breads, pastas, fruits, starchy vegetables, and anything with sugar in it. Once the carbohydrates are ingested, the body rapidly breaks them down to sugars. To the body, a slice of white bread isn't much different from a piece of chocolate cake; they're both a type of simple sugar.

The low-carbohydrate, high-protein diets limit how many carbohydrates you eat each day but encourage you to consume generous quantities of protein and are fairly liberal about the amount of fat you can take in. Essentially, these diets work because the absence of carbohydrates and an overall reduction in calories force the body to break down its fat stores for energy. Also, insulin hormone levels are suppressed. This results in relatively rapid weight loss for many people. In theory, it appears to be a faster weight-loss method than a normal low-calorie diet because the lack of carbohydrate calories—the preferred fuel for the body—generates a more efficient breakdown of fat.

As we discussed earlier, most overweight women with PCOS have elevated insulin levels. *Insulin is released by the pancreas mainly in response to carbohydrates.* By reducing carbohydrates or combining them with other foods (proteins or fats), women with PCOS can lower their insulin levels very effectively. In addition to being a quick and effective method of weight loss, these low-carbohydrate, high-protein diets are especially effective in restoring normal ovarian function to these women when their insulin levels drop. Insulin directly and indirectly stimulates testosterone production by the ovaries. For this reason, women may also find that their acne and unwanted hair growth lessen on these diets.

What If You Want to Try a Low-Carbohydrate, High-Protein Diet?

As you are probably well aware, there are a number of best-selling diet books that promote a low-carbohydrate, high-protein diet, and I suggest you browse the shelves of your local bookstore or an Internet bookseller for one of them. Some of the most popular low-carbohydrate, high-protein diet books include *The Dr. Atkins' Diet* series, *The Carbohydrate Addict's Diet* series, The *Zone* series, and *Protein Power and Sugar Busters!*

There are some basic guidelines common to all diets that share this strategy. First you must know the carbohydrate content in all of the foods you consume. Read the package of everything you buy to see the grams of carbohydrate in a serving. Consider purchasing a food guide that lists the protein, fat, and carbohydrate makeup of the foods that don't come packaged, such as fresh fruits and vegetables.

In general, these diets allow you to eat generous portions of meats and many vegetables. Keep in mind that fruits are almost entirely carbohydrate, but some fruits, like strawberries, have fewer grams of carbohydrate than others. Certain vegetables, such as potatoes, corn, carrots, tomatoes, peas, onions, and beans, have a significant amount of carbohydrates, so they must be minimized. Be careful in adding condiments or breading to your foods. Many of these diet books use the concept of a glycemic index to determine which carbohydrates are better than others. The glycemic index indicates how quickly carbohydrates are absorbed and how quickly the blood-sugar levels rise after a meal. A carbohydrate with a high glycemic index would be quickly absorbed, causing a rapid rise in blood-sugar levels. In response to rapid rises in blood-sugar levels, the pancreas releases large amounts of insulin. So some carbohydrates (those with a low glycemic index) are better in terms of how they influence insulin levels.

Low-carbohydrate, high-protein dieters report to me that they don't feel hungry between meals because they are eating fairly normal portions of food. It probably also has to do with the fact that protein and fat tend to be more filling than carbohydrates, and they take longer to digest. Another benefit these dieters report is that they don't seem to get the post-lunch or post-dinner drowsiness they experienced as a result of their previous eating habits.

Many of the popular diet books I mentioned restrict carbohydrates so completely that your body enters a starvation state called ketoacidosis. Ketoacids are breakdown products of fat metabolism; they build up in the bloodstream when no carbohydrates are available. However, the ketoacids may not be safe during an early pregnancy. For this reason I don't suggest that you actually become pregnant while in ketoacidosis. *Complete your dieting before trying to conceive.* Also, take a prenatal vitamin while dieting. This way, if you do inadvertently become pregnant, you're not at higher risk for birth defects.

What Does a Low-Carbohydrate, High-Protein Diet Look Like?

Here is a sample diet for a single day to give you an idea of what a low-carbohydrate, high-protein diet looks like. Notice that carbohydrates are not completely removed from the diet, and this sample is from a particularly restrictive diet. The best-selling low-carbohydrate, high-protein diet books will take you meal by meal in great detail through an entire diet using their own unique strategies. Many of the diet books have different stages or phases of carbohydrate restriction or offer intermittent "normal" meals to add back some carbohydrates and give you variety. Once again, *it's always best to be evaluated by your physician before beginning a diet.* These low-carbohydrate, high-protein diets may not be safe for women with certain medical problems, including kidney disease.

Breakfast: Scrambled cheese eggs
               Bacon

Multivitamin
A small glass of orange juice (or grapefruit juice)
and an extra large glass of water

Lunch: Chef's salad
An extra large glass of water or sugar-free drink

Snack: Deviled egg (or boiled egg), or cottage cheese, or
cheese, or beef jerky, or pickles, or peanuts
Any extra-large sugar-free drink

Dinner: A generous portion of steak
A large tossed salad, and/or vegetables (examples:
asparagus, mushrooms, cauliflower, peppers, sum-
mer squash, cucumber—all with plenty of butter)
Sugar-free gelatin with ½ cup strawberries
Any extra-large sugar-free drink

For women with PCOS who are within the normal BMI
range but have irregular menstrual cycles, dieting for weight loss
is probably not an effective treatment. However, consuming a
modified high-protein, low-carbohydrate diet with the intention
to reduce insulin levels while maintaining weight may be effective. If you find yourself in this group, I recommend a visit to
your obstetrician/gynecologist or a reproductive endocrinologist.

Five Vital Components for Weight Loss

1. Raising Your Metabolic Rate

The metabolic rate, which determines the number of calories
burned in a day, decreases about 2 percent per year starting at
age 18. This is one reason why we tend to gain weight over
time even if we eat the same things. One very unfair aspect of
obesity is that an increase in weight does not lead to a propor-
tional increase in the metabolic rate. This means that as a person gets heavier, losing weight becomes more difficult. It is

paradoxical but true that obese people need proportionately fewer calories as they get larger.

The most effective way to combat this lowering of the basal metabolic rate with age and weight is to combine caloric restriction with exercise. *Exercise is absolutely critical for successful weight loss.* Exercise not only burns calories, but it also suppresses appetite. It also raises the metabolic rate for 24 to 48 hours, continuing to burn calories long after the exercise is completed. Without this rise in the metabolic rate from exercise, weight loss is painfully slow and many women will eventually lose motivation and quit dieting. As with dieting, it is always recommended that you get evaluated by your physician if you intend to begin an exercise program.

> You have to burn 3,500 calories in order to lose one pound of weight. If you only skip desserts each day, assuming that a dessert with both lunch and dinner adds about 500 calories, it will take 210 days (about seven months) to lose 30 pounds. Unless you severely restrict calories or combine moderate caloric restriction with regular exercise, you can expect weight loss to be a very slow process. On the other hand, eating 250 calories more than you need each day—the number of calories in an average dessert item or candy bar—will result in an extra 25 pounds gained over one year.

2. Reaching Your Optimal Heart Rate

Any effective exercise program must include enough aerobic exercise to reach and maintain your optimal heart rate. Exercising inadequately will not raise your metabolic rate to the same degree, and you will find it more difficult to lose weight. *You should get regular exercise at least every other day and raise your pulse to the optimal level for 30 minutes during each session.* For an otherwise healthy woman, you can calculate your optimal heart rate by taking your age and subtracting it from 220, then taking 70 percent of that number. The final number represents the heartbeats per minute that you should reach and sustain during the aerobic exercise, which I refer to as your optimal target heart rate.

It doesn't matter what you decide to do for exercise. Choose an activity you enjoy and can do at least every other day year-round. Be sure that you bring your heart rate up to your optimal rate for at least 30 minutes during each exercise session. Don't get discouraged. You will need to build your exercise tolerance slowly over time, so don't expect to be able to do a full 30 minutes of exercise at your first session. It may take months for you to be able to reach and maintain your optimal heart rate during exercise.

Target Heart Rate During Exercise:

$$(220 - \text{your age}) \times 0.7 = \text{Optimal Heart Rate}$$

Example: If you are 30 years old, then $(220 - 30) \times 0.7 = 133$ beats per minute

---

3. Losing Weight with Friends

Experts in weight loss also suggest that you lose weight with group support. Try to find a group or another individual, such as your spouse or just a friend or two, to exercise with. This will make it more fun and will help you maintain your motivation. *It's crucial to have someone encouraging you and at the same time going through the process with you.* You can also join a formal group such as Overeaters Anonymous, if you feel you would benefit from a structured support group.

4. Maintaining Good Nutrition While Dieting

Don't think that just because your periods may be absent or irregular now, you don't have to worry about becoming pregnant. Overweight women who are dieting often become pregnant inadvertently due to the fertility-enhancing effects of their weight loss. For many overweight women with irregular menstrual periods, a modest amount of weight loss is all they need to trigger a resumption of ovulation and menstrual periods. I recommend to all my patients not to try to get pregnant until after they have finished their weight loss, but if you should accidentally become pregnant while dieting you'll want to ensure the health of your baby. *Make sure you are eating a healthy diet while you lose weight.* (See Chapter 7 for more details.)

All women should start taking a prenatal vitamin preconceptionally, but women dieting have an even greater chance of not getting enough vitamins and minerals in their diet. This puts their babies at higher risk for nutrition-related birth defects.

What if you're overweight but your menstrual cycles are normal, indicating that your fertility is probably intact? For general health reasons, and to decrease the risk of miscarriage and maternal pregnancy complications, many overweight women with regular periods will still want to lose weight prior to the pregnancy. If you find yourself in this group, it is very important that you maintain proper preconceptional nutritional requirements.

5. Being Realistic About Weight Loss

Above all, be patient! Think how many years it took to get to your present weight. It is unreasonable to think it will all come off in a few months. A five-pound weight loss in the first month and a loss of 20 to 30 pounds over four to five months is average. Additionally, as the pounds are shed subsequent weight loss becomes harder. The first ten to twenty pounds are the easiest to lose. For many of my patients successful weight loss is one of the most difficult things they have ever done. Don't give up!

Medications to Help You Ovulate If Weight Loss Is Unsuccessful

If weight loss after a prolonged effort is not successful, don't despair. You will want to schedule an appointment with your doctor to investigate further. After you have been fully evaluated, if other problems are ruled out and excessive weight appears to be the cause of your irregular menstrual cycles, your doctor will probably give you the choice of making one last effort to lose weight or using medications to help you ovulate.

Even if your menstrual periods don't return after weight loss and you end up needing medications to help you conceive, whatever weight you do lose will help the prescription medications to be more effective and make the pregnancy safer. If needed, there are other safe and effective prescription medications that can help you ovulate.

Metformin (trade name is Glucophage) is an insulin-sensitizing (-lowering) medication first developed for diabetes treatment. Over the last five to ten years it has become popular and widely utilized in women with PCOS to normalize menstrual cycles, facilitate ovulation, and to promote weight loss. Unlike other medications, such as clomiphene citrate (see below) or gonadotropins (FSH), metformin does not increase the risk of multiple pregnancy. It appears to work in a more natural way to normalize the balance of hormones and allow cycles to resume in some women. For all these reasons metformin has become a first-line treatment to consider.

Because this book focuses on ways to help yourself get pregnant naturally—without fertility medications—I will only mention one other very common medication to help you ovulate.

A widely used type of oral medication is an ovulation-induction agent called clomiphene citrate (Clomid [Hoechst Marion Roussel], clomiphene citrate tablets [Teva], or Serophene [Serono]). It is sometimes used by itself but often in combination with metformin if metformin alone was not able to normalize ovulation. Clomiphene citrate is a common medication that has been prescribed for decades. The main risk associated is a 5 to 10 percent chance of twins.

UNDERWEIGHT

Many American women would like to reach a body type that is thinner than they should be. The "in" look these days comes awfully close to anorexia, as typified by many of the models you see in magazines or actresses on popular television shows. The effort to achieve this level of thinness may induce women to maintain a BMI below 20, and this often leads to rare or absent menstrual periods. Female athletes are another group at high risk of menstrual irregularities due, in part, to extreme thinness.

Irregular menses usually indicates that ovulation is not occurring frequently or predictably, and the woman's fertility is compromised. Complete absence of menstrual periods assures infertility. Also, in terms of general medical concerns, estrogen levels in this group of women are often critically low, putting them at risk for early osteoporosis and accelerated heart disease.

The relationship between low body weight and fertility has been studied in detail by many investigators. Some authors have supported a theory that the amount of body weight and body fat are the key determinants of menstrual regularity and fertility. Dr. Rose E. Frisch, a well-known author on this topic from the Harvard School of Public Health, has proposed a critical weight and body-fat requirement for regular menstrual cycling. Dr. Frisch estimated that *22 percent body fat is the cutoff below which most women develop irregular menstrual cycles*. When a woman falls below this cutoff, her menstrual cycles often cease to be regular and in many women ovarian function will stop altogether. The 22 percent body fat is an approximate number, and some women are more or less sensitive to their body-fat levels.

Subsequent research has shown that, like absolute weight or BMI, body fat is not the whole explanation. Many other factors contribute to causing problems with the reproductive system, such as nutrition and psychological or physical stress. Nevertheless, the correlation between weight, body fat, and menstrual function does exist and is an important factor to consider.

How Does Being Underweight Cause Problems?

In evolutionary terms, the ability for the brain to recognize the level of fat in the body was probably an important advantage. In this way the brain could shut down unnecessary systems during a period of food shortage, when fat stores would diminish. During a period of inadequate caloric intake or actual starvation, it makes sense that the body wouldn't waste energy on the reproductive system, and a baby wouldn't be born when the mother might have difficulty nursing.

As we saw above in the discussion on overweight women, the brain assesses the amount of fat in the body by measuring levels of insulin and leptin in the bloodstream. In essence, the fat talks to the brain through these hormones, telling it when its stores are low. There is also good evidence that the ovaries respond to leptin and insulin levels in the bloodstream, so these hormones can directly affect the proper function of the ovaries. Therefore, fat stores directly influence the two main tissues involved in reproduction—the brain and the ovaries.

In response to leptin, insulin, and numerous other hormones and neurotransmitters, the brain shuts down the reproductive system in underweight women by stopping the flow of regulatory hormones to the ovaries. Normally, a part of the brain called the hypothalamus controls ovarian function. But in many underweight women the hypothalamus becomes inactive. When this happens the ovaries receive no stimulation, and they stop most of their functions. They produce little or no hormones, and ovulation and menstrual cycles become infrequent or cease altogether.

Other Important Issues for Underweight Women

There is another important problem that underweight women need to be aware of. If an underweight woman conceives she puts her baby at much higher risk for being significantly underweight at birth. Underweight babies are at higher risk for complications, similar to premature babies of equal size. This outcome can be improved by good maternal weight gain during the pregnancy, but *I strongly recommend that you normalize your weight before attempting to conceive.*

It is also important to mention that underweight women with infrequent or absent menstrual periods may face other significant health issues outside of pregnancy. As I mentioned earlier, lack of estrogen leads to bone density loss that will eventually result in osteoporosis. If this continues for a long time, the brittle bones reach a point where they fracture easily. I have two very thin college-age patients—one is a ballet dancer and the other is a long-distance runner—who have each suffered nontraumatic fractures of their bones: one had a hip fracture and the other had a fracture in her spine. Excessive exercise and inadequate caloric intake resulted in the suppression of the reproductive system, which in turn led to low estrogen levels, osteoporosis, and finally, broken bones. Excessively thin women are also at higher risk for miscarriage through the development of luteal phase deficiency. This problem is reviewed in more detail in the exercise section of this chapter.

What Can Be Done If You Are Underweight?

Clearly, *if you have irregular or absent menstrual periods and you find yourself in the "underweight" range on the BMI graph, you need to seriously consider gaining some weight.* The most common problem I encounter with my underweight patients is that they don't want to believe me when I tell them they are underweight. Our society's warped sense of ideal weight, combined with an inability for many women to accurately assess their own body image, conspire to make many women deny what is often very obvious to any bystander. For these reasons, I keep a BMI chart in my office and have the patient plot herself on the graph to convince her firsthand that she is too thin.

The solution is very obvious although quite difficult for many excessively thin women to accept. Even if I succeed in persuading a patient she is underweight, I usually encounter a lot of resistance to the notion that her weight is the cause of her lack of menstrual periods. Some women may respond that a friend who is even thinner than they are had no trouble conceiving. These women don't realize that the body's natural response to low fat stores may differ among individuals. I often have little success in motivating this group of women to gain any weight in order to see if this will correct the problem. As you would imagine, convincing a competitive runner or balle-rina that she needs to gain weight and reduce her activity is difficult. However, even thin women who are not athletes or dancers have usually worked very hard to get themselves to their present weight and are resistant to suggestions to gain any weight.

If an underweight woman with infrequent or absent men-strual periods wants to become pregnant, then weight gain and reduced activity are the most natural solutions. Depending on how severe the situation, gaining as little as 5 percent of a woman's present weight may help. For example, a six-pound weight gain for a woman weighing 120 pounds may be all that is needed to resume menses and reestablish normal fertility. Often my patients can remember what weight they were when they previously had normal menstrual periods. This weight then becomes the target weight to achieve. A woman may have to continue to gain weight until her BMI is greater than 20 or her body fat percentage is greater than 22 percent before menstrual cycles normalize.

There are injectable medications, called gonadotropins, that are very successful in causing ovulation in this group of women, but these should be considered for treatment only af-ter conservative measures have failed, due to the risks, side ef-fects, and expense involved. When an underweight woman with rare or absent periods is not trying to get pregnant, she should talk with her physician about taking supplemental es-trogen to protect her bones and heart.

Figure 6.4
ANOREXIA NERVOSA

Anorexia nervosa is a serious problem that results in extreme thinness and lack of menstrual periods. It is crucial to identify women with this disorder because as many as 10 percent of affected women will die from the disease. Following are the major characteristics of anorexia nervosa:

1. Lack of menstrual periods
2. Onset of these problems between age 10 and 30
3. Weight loss of 25 percent, or weight at least 15 percent below normal for age and height
4. Special attitudes:
   a. Distorted body image (unable to see oneself as too thin)
   b. Denial of any problem
   c. Unusual handling or hoarding of food
5. At least one of the following:
   a. Slow heartbeat (usually below 60 beats per minute)
   b. Overactivity (excessive exercise despite being too thin)
   c. Episodes of overeating or bingeing (bulimia)
   d. Vomiting or excessive laxative use (purging)
   e. Excessive growth of thin hairs (lanugo) in normally non-hairy areas
6. No other known medical or psychiatric problem that could be the cause
7. Other common findings (but not required for the diagnosis):
   a. Constipation
   b. Orange skin or the whites of the eyes (hypercarotenemia)
   c. Low blood pressure
   d. Excessive drinking of water

EXERCISE AND FERTILITY

The recognition that excessive exercise can influence a woman's reproductive health is not new. In the first century A.D., Soranus of Ephesus wrote a book called *On the Diseases of Women.* In it he noted that lack of menstrual periods was frequently observed in women who took too much exercise.

Only recently has female participation in sports become accepted and encouraged. It wasn't until 1966 that a woman, Roberta Gibb, first ran in the Boston Marathon. In fact, Roberta Gibb ran unofficially, and it was not until 1972 that the Boston Athletic Association, organizers of the Boston Marathon, allowed women to enter the race. In that same year, Congress passed Title IX of the Educational Assistance Act to force college athletic departments to treat female athletes equally to male athletes.

The passage of Title IX was a key event in the modern age of female athletics. Increased opportunities for women's athletics programs generated many more female college athletes. The increased numbers of female college athletes, combined with society's validation of female athletics, encouraged a large number of women to exercise. There has also been nothing less than a "fitness craze" that started in the 1970s and continues to influence our society today.

In this section I will review why and how reproductive functions can change in response to exercise, and when a woman may encounter problems if she exercises excessively. Women who exercise too much have a lot in common with underweight women in terms of their reduction in fertility, due mostly to irregularities in the menstrual cycle and ovulation. These women are also at higher risk for miscarriage. I will offer recommendations to maximize fertility and decrease the risk of miscarriage associated with exercise.

Do not misunderstand my message. In general, regular moderate exercise is very healthy and often fertility-enhancing. I am a strong proponent of regular exercise in reproductive-age women. It is only excessive exercise that can reduce fertility. The most common problem initially is a subtle shortening of the menstrual cycles with the associated hormonal problem, luteal phase deficiency (we'll discuss more about luteal phase deficiency further along). Next, the intervals between menstrual periods start to lengthen, with irregular or absent ovulation. Eventually a woman may progress to a complete lack of menstrual periods (amenorrhea).

If your menstrual periods become short, unpredictable, or absent, then your chances for getting pregnant are obviously lower. The good news is that, *in nearly all cases, any changes related to exercise are completely reversible, and there is no permanent effect on fertility.*

Just Do It?

Much of the research on exercise and menstrual change has involved runners, but it probably applies to most other types of intense exercise as well. It is estimated that over half of the serious runners who still have menstrual periods have abbreviated cycles that are either not ovulatory, despite apparently regular intervals of bleeding, or are deficient in the hormone progesterone. Inadequate progesterone can lead to decreased fertility and a higher risk of miscarriage. This means that a large number of women who exercise heavily and are menstruating still may suffer from decreased fertility and a higher risk of miscarriage without realizing it.

It has been difficult to determine specific guidelines for runners' mileage or intensity to prevent menstrual changes. This is because each female athlete differs in many respects, including body fat, weight, overall fitness, training schedule, training intensity, and nutrition. Other proposed contributing factors include the effect of elevated body temperature on the ovaries, stress on the mind and body, inadequate protein and caloric intake, and alteration of the normal pattern of hormones released by the brain (such as the natural release of opiates during exercise, called the "runner's high").

A few studies have shown a significant relationship between the weekly mileage run and menstrual or ovulatory irregularities. Some authors have proposed absolute mileage cutoffs for female runners to help prevent menstrual or ovulatory irregularities. Research by Dr. Ralph Hale and colleagues at the University of Hawaii has suggested that 20 miles per week is the level where menstrual changes occur in many women.

Most likely the causes for exercise-induced menstrual cycle changes are many, and the problem may not be solved by merely gaining a few pounds or eating a better diet or running 19 instead of 22 miles per week. Common sense dictates that whether you exercise or not, if you have irregular or absent menstrual periods and you find yourself in the "underweight" range on the BMI graph or with less than 22 percent body fat, you need to seriously consider gaining some weight.

In my own personal experience working with college athletes, the cause for the irregular periods is not always clear. For instance, many of the young women don't have abnormally low body-fat percentages or high-mileage workouts. The physical and mental stress of competitive athletics may be one of the most important factors for changes in the menstrual cycle. Even among the very thin and low body-fat athletes, merely going home for the winter or summer break can often bring back the menstrual periods within a few weeks, even before the women have had a chance to gain much weight.

Exercise and Miscarriage

My wife, Kara, was training for a marathon up until a few weeks before our first attempt to get pregnant. Although we conceived on our first try, this pregnancy ended in an early miscarriage. A few days after the loss, my wife asked me whether I thought the marathon training could have had anything to do with the miscarriage. I told her that I wasn't sure, but I would see what research had been done on that question.

There are a number of studies that show a higher miscarriage risk in athletes due to the phenomenon called luteal phase deficiency. Luteal phase deficiency is also a cause of decreased fertility. What exactly is this condition? The second half of the menstrual cycle is referred to as the luteal phase, and this is when the hormone progesterone is produced in large amounts (see Chapter 1). As we have noted, while estrogen stimulates the lining of the uterus to thicken during the first half of the menstrual cycle, progesterone—produced after ovulation—has the vital role of preparing the uterine lining for pregnancy. Insufficient progesterone production leads to a poorly prepared uterine lining that cannot adequately support the embryo when it tries to implant or grow. Luteal phase deficiency describes these low progesterone levels and the inadequate uterine lining that can result.

A study published in the *New England Journal of Medicine* by Dr. B. A. Bullen and colleagues at Boston University evaluated 28 women not in training who had normal menstrual cycles. Over a one-month period the women gradually increased their daily running mileage from four miles per day to ten miles per day. These women were found to have a 33 percent incidence of luteal phase deficiency if they maintained their normal weight during the month, and a 63 percent incidence if any weight was lost. The results of this study impressively illustrate that women who exercise intensively are at higher risk for luteal phase deficiency and the associated decrease in fertility and increase in miscarriage rates.

How to Recognize Luteal Phase Deficiency Yourself

Luteal phase deficiency frequently results in menstrual cycles that are shorter than normal, but often this is so subtle that it's difficult for a woman to notice. Regardless of the total length of your cycle, what almost all women have in common is that the luteal phase of the cycle should last about 14 days. If you use an ovulation-prediction kit, add 14 days to the day of your positive urinary test and that should coincide with the last day of your cycle. If the time from the positive test to the last day of your cycle is 12 days or less, this means your luteal phase is abnormally short and you may have luteal phase deficiency. Using a basal-body-temperature chart (BBT), if your menstrual bleeding begins less than 11 days after the rise in your basal body temperature then this might also indicate luteal phase deficiency.

If you believe you may have luteal phase deficiency, especially if you have had a previous miscarriage, you should consult your obstetrician/gynecologist. You should consider decreasing your amount and intensity of exercise and gaining some weight (if applicable); this will probably solve your problem.

Could this luteal phase deficiency be the explanation for my wife's first miscarriage, or was it just bad luck? It is quite variable due to age, but in general, miscarriage occurs in at least 25 percent of all pregnancies. So, the odds are it was probably not LPD, but we'll never know for sure. If you exercise, especially if you have noticed any menstrual irregularities, it would be prudent for you to consider not only the possibility of changing your weight and diet, but also altering your exercise routine to reduce the chance of miscarriage.

Neither the college athletes that I work with, nor my wife's friends who are avid runners, appreciate those suggestions. Unfortunately, many women who exercise intensely will have to accept the fact that at some point they will have to decrease the amount or intensity of exercise, either to become pregnant or because they are pregnant. Additionally, athletes are at risk for insufficient protein, iron, and zinc consumption, and these deficiencies can reduce fertility. Nutritional concerns are discussed in more detail in Chapter 7.

How to Change Your Exercise Routine

Making specific exercise recommendations is difficult because each woman is so unique. If your menstrual periods are irregular or absent (greater than three months without menstrual bleeding) then I recommend that you make an appointment with your obstetrician/gynecologist. If you are an avid runner and your menstrual cycles are short or irregular, and you are concerned about the possibility of luteal phase deficiency, I suggest you decrease your daily mileage by 25 percent or run less than 20 miles per week. Do not run every day. Try reducing your pace by at least 10 percent (for example, 7:30 minutes per mile would become 8:15 minutes per mile), as a reasonable way to decrease the intensity. Women who participate in other sports, such as swimming or aerobics, should also reduce their distance and time by a significant percentage, exercise less frequently, and reduce the speed or intensity of their workout by at least 10 percent. If underweight, female athletes should keep in mind the recommendations given earlier in this chapter.

Female athletes must consider the fact that muscle weighs more than fat. This means that even though many female athletes may not be underweight on standard BMI charts, their body-fat percentage is often still too low. *Remember, for normal fertility it is important not only that your BMI be approximately 20 or higher, but also that you have a body-fat percentage of at least 22.* Use Figure 6.2 to determine your body-fat percentage; if you find it is too low, you should consider gaining weight regardless of your place on the BMI chart.

To illustrate some of the issues related to both decreased fertility and increased risk of miscarriage, I'll once again refer to my wife's situation. Before trying to get pregnant a second time, Kara had many questions about how her exercise level might impact on the next pregnancy. Should she decrease her mileage? If so, by how much? What about gaining some weight?

With our second pregnancy we decided Kara would decrease her mileage from about 20 miles per week to about 15 miles per week, and she would gain some weight. We settled on a weight gain of six pounds because that would get her back to her previous weight before she began the oral contraceptives and heavy training. She also agreed to decrease her pace. We hoped that these changes in her training and weight might help prevent menstrual and ovulatory irregularities, as well as preventing luteal phase deficiency, which may have caused the previous miscarriage. She also started a prenatal vitamin and increased her protein intake two months before we started trying to conceive.

What were our results? We got pregnant on our first try and it resulted in our wonderful son, Scott. So many things go into having a healthy baby that it's difficult to say whether our plan was helpful or not, but I'd like to think it was.

If these suggestions do not help normalize your menstrual cycles within a two- or three-month period, I would suggest you consult your physician. Athletes are just as likely as anyone else to have other potentially serious problems that can cause irregular menstrual cycles. If your cycles are completely normal despite your exercise level, then you probably don't need to make any alterations.

CONCLUSIONS

Weight and exercise are issues that affect a large number of readers. Perhaps the most important thing is to be able to recognize when you are in a high-risk group and understand the importance of optimizing your weight or exercise regimen for your health and the health of your baby. If identified and accepted, the majority of these issues can be optimized on your own without the need for any formal medical care. *By normalizing your weight and applying some common sense to your exercise routine you can dramatically improve your fertility, decrease your risks and the risks to your baby during pregnancy, and reduce your chances of miscarriage.* See Figure 6.5 for a summary chart to help you organize all of the recommendations that might apply to you.

Figure 6.5
SUMMARY

Weight

BMI Calculation (Plot yourself on Figure 6.1, page 127)
1. You are underweight if your BMI is less than 20
2. You are overweight if your BMI is greater than 25

Body Fat Calculation (See Figure 6.2, page 129)
In general, your body fat percentage should be greater than or equal to 22 and less than 28.

Overweight
You are at higher risk for irregular menstrual periods, complications during pregnancy, and miscarriage.
1. General weight loss strategies
   a. Restrict your intake of calories. Choose a diet that you believe you can stick to for at least six months.

   b. Exercise for 30 minutes at your optimal heart rate at least every other day of the week. (Optimal heart rate=[220− your age]×0.7).

   c. Lose weight and exercise with group support—at least with a friend or your spouse.

2. Have realistic expectations about the time frame required to lose the weight. A five-pound weight loss in the first month and a loss of 20 to 30 pounds over four to five months is average.

3. Women with polycystic ovarian syndrome (PCOS)

   a. Exercise using the guidelines listed above.

   b. Institute whatever diet you think best fits your eating habits/personality. If you have no idea, consider trying a high-protein, low-carbohydrate diet. (Many best-selling diet books are available at your local bookstore.)

   c. Use the guidelines for general weight loss listed above.

   d. See Chapter 7 for additional information on diet and PCOS.

Underweight

If you have short, irregular, or absent menstrual periods:

1. Gain at least the number of pounds that equals 5 percent of your ideal body weight (for example, a six-pound weight gain for a woman who should weigh about 125 pounds). If not successful, gain the number of pounds required to bring your BMI up to 20.

2. Consider increasing your body-fat percentage above 22 percent.

3. Take a multivitamin daily.

4. Assure dietary protein consumption of at least 60 grams per day.

5. Even if you have normal menstrual cycles, consider gaining weight until your body mass index (BMI) is greater than 20

in order to reduce the chances that your baby will have complications due to being underweight at birth.

Exercise

If your menstrual periods are short, irregular, or absent, and you exercise heavily:

1. If you are underweight, follow the recommendations in the section on being underweight. Whether you are underweight or not, consider reducing the duration and intensity of exercise:

   a. If you are a long-distance runner, consider reducing daily mileage by 25 percent, or running less than 20 miles per week. Do not exercise every day. (Other sports will require corresponding reductions of at least 25 percent in duration of activity.)

   b. If you run, decrease your pace by at least 10 to 20 percent. (Other sports will require equivalent analogous changes in intensity of exercise.)

2. Consider that muscle weighs more than fat; you may be in the normal BMI range but still have too low a percentage of body fat. Gain weight until your body fat is at least 22 percent.

3. If you keep a menstrual calendar and you note that your menstrual bleeding begins 12 days or less after your positive ovulation-prediction kit result, or less than 11 days after your rise in basal body temperature, then you may be at increased risk for miscarriage or reduced fertility (see discussion of luteal phase deficiency).

7

Diet and Nutrition

To bring on the menses, recover the flesh with puddings, roast meats, a good wine, fresh air, and sun.
—*Gilman Thompson,* Practical Dietetics, *1847*

THE influence of diet on reproductive health has been recognized for centuries. Charles Darwin, the same scientist who proposed the theory of evolution, noted that animals with good nutrition and a plentiful food supply are more fertile. Chapter 3 focused on the prevention of birth defects through good nutrition. In the previous chapter, dieting with the intention to lose weight was reviewed. In this chapter, I will evaluate the effects of your nutrition and everyday diet on fertility and miscarriage.

There is no doubt that nutrition plays a vital role in reproduction. Deficiencies in iron, zinc, and vitamin C, excessive caffeine consumption, alcohol consumption, and inadequate protein or daily caloric intake have all been implicated in reducing fertility. Some of these factors may also affect the chance of miscarriage. Recently there has been a lot of excitement about reports that taking an aspirin a day will improve fertility. Some researchers have suggested special diets or nutritional supplementation for women with common gynecological problems such as fibroids, endometriosis, or polycystic ovarian syndrome. By the end of this chapter, you will understand how to maximize your diet to become pregnant faster and have a successful outcome to your pregnancy.

CAFFEINE

The average American drinks more than 30 gallons of caffeinated coffee each year. Caffeine is found in many other products, including chocolate, over-the-counter and prescription medications, tea, diet pills, and soft drinks. A few studies have looked at caffeine intake and time to conception. There appears to be a relationship between the amount of caffeine a woman consumes and a delay in becoming pregnant. However, the amount of caffeine it takes to have an effect on fertility, and how significant this effect actually is, have not been established.

There is a much stronger association with decreased fertility when a woman *drinks alcohol in addition to caffeinated beverages*. As you might imagine, it is difficult to study the isolated effect of caffeine on reproduction because so many other environmental factors may be involved. Based on the preliminary data, I would suggest you eliminate your caffeine intake before trying to get pregnant—if you want to conceive as rapidly as possible.

Figure 7.1
CAFFEINE CONTENT OF COMMON PRODUCTS

Coffee (per 8 ounces):

Regular coffee	80–280 milligrams (depending on strength)
Decaffeinated coffee	4–8 milligrams

Soft Drinks (per 12 ounces):

Coca-Cola, Pepsi	35–45 milligrams
Mountain Dew	54 milligrams

Tea (per 8 ounces):

Instant tea	40–80 milligrams (depending on strength)
Brewed tea	16–160 milligrams (depending on strength)
Iced tea (per 12 ounces)	75 milligrams

Other:

Hot chocolate (per 8 ounces)	8–36 milligrams
Chocolate candy bar (2 ounces)	up to 30 milligrams
Excedrin (per tablet)	65 milligrams
Cold medications (per tablet)	15–30 milligrams

ALCOHOL

Most women know that drinking alcohol during pregnancy is a bad idea. Few women realize that alcohol should be stopped before trying to get pregnant because it can reduce fertility. In a study by Rosemarie Hakim, Ph.D., and colleagues from Johns Hopkins University, published in 1998, nondrinkers had a 25 percent chance of getting pregnant each month (the normal expected probability), while women who drank one alcoholic beverage per week had a 17 percent chance of getting pregnant, and women who drank anywhere between one and seven drinks per week had a 12 percent chance of getting pregnant. Therefore, the results of this study indicate that *one alcoholic beverage per week will reduce your fertility by about one-third, and more than one drink per week could reduce your chances by more than 50 percent.*

Interestingly, this study also showed that drinking both alcohol and caffeine exacerbates the fertility-reducing effects of each. My own recommendation is to stop drinking alcoholic beverages at least one month before starting your attempts to conceive.

AN ASPIRIN A DAY KEEPS
THE FERTILITY SPECIALIST AWAY?

A study published in the spring of 1999 by a group of Argentine fertility specialists created an enormous amount of interest around the use of low-dose aspirin to promote fertility. The results of that study indicated a dramatic increase in pregnancy rates among women who took a low-dose aspirin a day compared to taking a placebo (inactive) pill each day. Many fertility experts have questioned the validity of these results. This section will summarize the information available to answer the question of whether women should use aspirin to increase their chances of getting pregnant.

Only a few studies have been undertaken to address this question. The study by the Argentine group in 1999 had the women take 100 milligrams of aspirin each day or an identical-appearing placebo pill. The results were astounding. Women who took the low dose of aspirin each day had a 45 percent chance of getting pregnant each in vitro fertilization (IVF) cycle, versus a 28 percent chance per cycle for the placebo group. The women in this study were all undergoing IVF treatment—a high-technology fertility therapy also referred to as having a "test tube baby"—to correct their documented infertility. For this reason aspirin treatment may not offer any benefit to ordinary couples attempting to conceive.

In contrast, Dr. Jerome Check and colleagues at the University of Medicine and Dentistry of New Jersey published a study in 1998 that evaluated the use of 81 milligrams of aspirin (the dose found in a "baby" aspirin) among a different group of infertile women. This study indicated that one of these aspirins each day did not improve the chances for pregnancy.

Despite the inconsistencies between the two most recent studies, the almost unbelievable increase in pregnancy success found in the Argentine study convinced a number of highly respected fertility programs in the United States and Europe to adopt the use of low-dose aspirin with all their IVF patients. The reasoning seems to be that even if the aspirin treatment proves ineffective in future studies, one low-dose aspirin a day shouldn't cause any harm. Unfortunately this is not entirely true, because aspirin taken during early pregnancy has been associated with a serious, though rare, birth defect.

Aspirin has been shown to increase the risk for gastroschisis, a birth defect of the fetal abdomen where the abdominal wall is not formed, thereby leaving the internal organs exposed. As you can imagine, this is a very serious birth defect. The best study of the relationship between aspirin and gastroschisis was published in 1996 by Dr. C. P. Torfs and colleagues from the California Birth Defects Monitoring Program. It found that *both aspirin and ibuprofen (the active ingredient in Motrin or Advil), but not acetaminophen (the active ingredient in Tylenol), showed a greater than fourfold increased risk for gastroschisis when mothers used these medications during the first trimester of pregnancy.*

I am skeptical that aspirin treatment would offer any benefit for the readers of this book. It would be easy for me to simply cite the latest study, showing a 60 percent increase in your chances of becoming pregnant by taking one low dose of aspirin a day. But as we've seen, it's not that simple. No study has ever evaluated whether ordinary couples can benefit from the use of preconceptional aspirin to promote fertility. Although gastroschisis is a rare birth defect associated with aspirin use preconceptionally or during early pregnancy, you should keep in mind that potential harm could result from the use of this drug in this setting.

CALORIC INTAKE

In Chapter 6 I reviewed in detail the reproductive problems associated with being underweight. If you are not consuming adequate calories to keep your weight and body fat in the normal range, there is a good chance your fertility will be reduced. Additionally, beginning and ending the pregnancy underweight can reduce fetal growth and increase the risk for neonatal complications.

If you are overweight, then dieting for weight loss prior to the pregnancy can increase your fertility and decrease the chance of miscarriage and pregnancy complications. Dieting isn't healthy during pregnancy, so weight loss should always be completed before you attempt to conceive. Keep in mind that weight loss in an overweight woman is often fertility enhancing. Use a form of birth control during the weight loss to assure you don't conceive before planned. I also recommend a daily prenatal multivitamin, so that in case you do conceive unexpectedly the risk of nutrition-related birth defects will be minimized.

PROTEIN

Inadequate protein intake can decrease the frequency of menstrual periods and may also contribute to early miscarriage.

The recommended protein consumption for nonpregnant women is at least 45 to 50 grams per day. Once pregnant, a woman needs to increase her protein intake to at least *60 to 65 grams per day.* Women who exercise will need to supplement their protein, along with other vitamins, minerals, and calories used during the exertion. Foods that are high in protein include meats, poultry, fish, dry beans and peas, soy products, eggs, cheese, cottage cheese, milk, and nuts (see Figure 7.2).

Figure 7.2
PROTEIN CONTENT OF COMMON FOODS

Lamb chop (3 ounces)	32 grams
Steak (3 ounces)	20 grams
Liver (3 ounces)	22 grams
Ham (3 ounces)	19 grams
Fish (3 ounces of haddock)	17 grams
Chicken (3 ounces)	26 grams
Milk (1 cup, any % milkfat)	8 grams
Cheese (American, 1 ounce)	6 grams
Cottage cheese (1 cup)	27 grams
Yogurt (plain, 8 ounces)	10 grams
Egg (one)	6 grams
Macaroni and cheese (1 cup)	10 grams
Cornmeal (1 cup)	11 grams
Rice (long-grain, 1 cup, cooked)	4 grams
Spaghetti (1 cup)	7 grams
Almonds (1 cup)	21 grams
Peanuts (1 cup)	37 grams
Navy beans (cooked, 1 cup)	15 grams
Black-eyed peas (cooked, 1 cup)	13 grams

Brussels sprouts (cooked, 1 cup)   7 grams
Broccoli (cooked, 1 cup)   6 grams

VITAMINS AND MINERALS

The nutritional requirements to reduce the chances of birth defects were discussed in detail in Chapter 3. Here I will review many of the other issues surrounding nutrition and reproduction. Certain vitamin and mineral deficiencies can decrease your fertility or increase your chance of miscarriage. We will also consider the sources of vitamins and minerals to use when correcting or preventing deficiencies.

Iron

It has been estimated that as many as one-third of all adult women are iron deficient. Some indirect evidence indicates that maternal anemia, caused by low iron levels, can result in decreased fertility, a higher risk of premature birth, and complications soon after birth. Of course, all women with iron-deficiency anemia should take action to correct this condition regardless of whether or not they're trying to get pregnant.

The daily recommended dose of iron is 60 milligrams (of elemental iron) per day preconceptionally and during pregnancy. Some good sources for iron include organ meats—liver in particular—peas, lean ground beef, prune juice, spinach, oysters, and beans; and to a lesser extent other meats and shellfish, eggs, nuts, dried fruit, and leafy green vegetables and, of course, a prenatal multivitamin (see Figure 7.3). Keep in mind that vitamin C improves the absorption of iron, so make sure you're getting adequate amounts of vitamin C along with the iron-containing foods.

Figure 7.3
COMMON DIETARY SOURCES OF IRON

Organ meats (4 ounces)	8–15 milligrams
Lean ground beef (4 ounces)	4 milligrams
Peas (1 cup)	6 milligrams
Prune juice (1 cup)	10 milligrams
Spinach (1 cup)	4 milligrams
Raisins (1 cup)	5 milligrams
Kidney beans (1 cup)	4.5 milligrams

Some women will need to take iron tablets daily if their anemia is severe. If additional supplementation is necessary, iron supplements are available over the counter or with your physician's prescription. When supplementing your diet with any mineral, you need to know how much "elemental" mineral is in each tablet. Iron, for example, is always bound, or chelated, to something else. The milligrams in each tablet do not usually equal the amount of elemental iron but rather a combination of the chelated substance and the iron, *so only a fraction of the total milligrams will be iron*. You'll have to check the label to determine how much elemental iron is present to make sure you are adequately supplementing. This mistake is most common with calcium supplements, so I'll return to this issue in the calcium section.

Zinc

Zinc is an essential nutrient in the normal growth of a baby. Maternal zinc deficiency may cause neurologic birth defects and can also result in decreased fertility and a higher rate of miscarriage. Zinc is not stored well in the body and therefore requires daily supplementation. *Preconceptionally and during pregnancy, a woman's zinc requirements increase to 25 milligrams daily.*

High-risk groups for zinc deficiency include heavy exercisers, vegetarians, and women who use oral contraceptives up until the time of conception. Exercise results in a significant loss of zinc through sweating. Heavy exercisers need to consider additional zinc supplementation above the recommended 25 milligrams a day in order to compensate for increased losses by the sweat glands.

Some foods that contain zinc in high concentrations are meats, such as liver, red meats, and seafood. Oysters are the single best source of zinc. Plants are very poor in terms of zinc concentration, and this presents a particular challenge for many vegetarians. However, I will review some plant sources for zinc a little later in this chapter. And as always, a vitamin supplement will solve your problem.

Figure 7.4

COMMON DIETARY SOURCES OF ZINC

Black-eyed peas (1 cup)	7 milligrams
Atlantic oysters (3 ounces)	63 milligrams
Beef or liver (3 ounces)	5 milligrams
Potato with skin (1 medium sized)	1 milligram
Macaroni (1 cup)	0.7 milligrams
Green peas (1 cup)	2 milligrams

Vitamin C

Vitamin C deficiency has been associated with decreased fertility, increased miscarriage, and preterm labor. It may be that vitamin C deficiency causes these problems indirectly through anemia, because it acts as a cofactor for iron absorption. The exact relationship is uncertain at the present time.

Vitamin C is one of the water-soluble vitamins, so it's not stored in the body for any length of time and needs to be supplemented daily. *The daily requirement for vitamin C preconceptionally is 65–80 milligrams.* You can find vitamin C in many fruits, such as citrus, strawberries, watermelon, and cantaloupe. Many vegetables are also good sources of vitamin C, including cauliflower, tomatoes, bean sprouts, and some leafy green vegetables. Vitamin C is destroyed by cooking, drying, and aging—so eat these vitamin C-rich foods fresh.

Figure 7.5
COMMON DIETARY SOURCES OF VITAMIN C

Orange juice (8 ounces)	60 milligrams
Orange (1)	65 milligrams
Cantaloupe (¼)	45 milligrams
Grapefruit (½)	44 milligrams
Liver (3 ounces)	23 milligrams
Apple (1)	6 milligrams
Avocado (½)	18 milligrams
Blueberries (1 cup)	20 milligrams

Folic Acid

In Chapter 3 we reviewed the vital importance for all women (with no special risk factors for brain or spinal cord malformations) to supplement 0.4 milligrams (400 micrograms) of folic acid a day preconceptionally in order to prevent birth defects. If you want to try to supplement your folic acid requirements with your diet, you have many options: leafy green vegetables, asparagus, broccoli, beans, lentils, dried peas, orange juice, and fortified breakfast cereals.

However, you must remember that dietary sources of folic acid are not as bioavailable, meaning that even if a helping of food contains a certain amount of folic acid, the body isn't able to use it all. In fact, you must consume twice as much dietary folic acid to equal the folic acid found in a vitamin pill or supplemented breakfast cereal. *This means that it takes food containing 0.8 milligrams of folic acid for the body to remove the 0.4 milligrams required each day.*

Because all the research studies have used folic acid in pill form to prevent neural tube defects, and because it is difficult to assess the exact amount of folic acid absorbed through diet, the Centers for Disease Control (CDC), the Institute of Medicine, and the U.S. Public Health Service recommend a vitamin supplement rather than a dietary source of folic acid.

Calcium—Consider the Source

To maximize fetal health and appropriate growth, *women who want to become pregnant should be getting 1,200 milligrams of calcium each day.* Although I am not aware of any fertility problems associated with low calcium levels prior to pregnancy, there are some potential adverse effects of calcium supplementation that you should keep in mind. These involve the type of calcium supplement you choose.

If you think you're not ingesting enough calcium and you decide to take a supplement, consider the source. It might seem that unpurified sources of calcium, like bone meal, oyster shell, or dolomite, would be more natural and therefore better for you. Unfortunately, *some of these natural sources can be contaminated with high levels of lead, arsenic, or mercury.* Clearly you don't want to expose yourself to these toxic contaminants preconceptionally or during pregnancy.

As I noted in the section on iron, keep in mind that when supplementing your diet with a mineral you are interested in how much "elemental" mineral is in each tablet. For example, a common brand of calcium citrate comes in 500 milligram tablets, but only about 100 milligrams of the tablet is actually elemental calcium. You would need five tablets to supplement 500 milligrams of calcium with this product. Calcium comes in many forms: calcium gluconate, calcium carbonate, calcium citrate, and others. Read the label to see how much elemental calcium is in each product.

I recommend taking Tums tablets, made of calcium carbonate (a common source of calcium). This is a safe and economical way to meet your calcium requirements. A 500-milligrams tablet of Tums has 200 milligrams of elemental calcium in it. Consider your normal diet to see approximately how many milligrams of calcium you are taking in each day, and then supplement the rest so that you're taking a total of 1,200 milligrams of elemental calcium a day.

Figure 7.6
COMMON DIETARY SOURCES OF CALCIUM

Milk (any % milkfat—one cup)	300 milligrams
American cheese (one slice)	210 milligrams
Turnip greens (⅔ cup)	200 milligrams
Tofu (3 ounces)	125 milligrams
Spinach (½ cup)	90 milligrams
Broccoli (½ cup)	70 milligrams
Peanuts (⅔ cup)	70 milligrams
Green beans (½ cup)	60 milligrams

OTHER VITAMINS/MINERALS

As we learn more about the role of nutrition in fertility and birth defects, new recommendations will surely arise. My advice to you would be that *until more is known about this subject, take a daily multivitamin (preferably one formulated as a "prenatal" product) with 400 to 600 micrograms of folic acid, and make sure the levels of other vitamins and minerals meet but do not exceed the recommended dietary allowances (or dietary reference intakes) for a pregnant woman* (see Figure 7.7).

There are many excellent over-the-counter products, so you don't necessarily need a prescription from your physician. However, your insurance will frequently cover medications obtained by a physician's prescription or charge you a modest copayment. If this applies to you, consider calling your doctor's office and asking for a prenatal vitamin prescription—it might save some money.

In general, it's very hard to consume toxic levels of vitamins and minerals in your diet. Usually the concerns are inadequate levels of vitamins and minerals from the foods you consume, or excessive vitamin and mineral supplementation through megadosing, as we reviewed in Chapter 3.

VEGETARIANS

Strict vegetarians are at a higher risk for birth defects and decreased fertility if they're not aware of their special needs for nutritional supplementation. Most importantly, vegetarians need to pay close attention to any nutritional deficiencies they may have. If vegetarians compensate for these deficiencies, their fertility should be normal and the risk for birth defects no different than that of nonvegetarians. Diet also appears to be a

Figure 7.7A

Dietary Reference Intakes to Apply Preconceptionally

Life-Stage Group	Calcium (mg/d)	Phosphorus (mg/d)	Magnesium (mg/d)	Vitamin D (μg/d)[a,b]	Fluoride (mg/d)	Thiamin (mg/d)	Riboflavin (mg/d)	Niacin (mg/d)[c]	Vitamin B6 (mg/d)	Folate (μg/d)[d]	Vitamin B12 (μg/d)	Pantothenic Acid (mg/d)	Biotin (μg/d)	Choline[e] (mg/d)
Pregnancy														
≤18 yr	1,300*	1,250	400	5*	3*	1.4	1.4	18	1.9	600[a,h]	2.6	6*	30*	450*
19–30 yr	1,000*	700	350	5*	3*	1.4	1.4	18	1.9	600[a,h]	2.6	6*	30*	450*
31–50 yr	1,000*	700	360	5*	3*	1.4	1.4	18	1.9	600[a,h]	2.6	6*	30*	450*

NOTE: This table presents Recommended Dietary Allowances (RDAs) in **bold type** and Adequate Intakes (AIs) in ordinary type followed by an asterisk (*). RDAs and AIs may both be used as goals for individual intake. RDAs are set to meet the needs of almost all (97 to 98 percent) individuals in a group. For healthy breastfed infants, the AI is the mean intake. The AI for other life-stage and gender groups is believed to cover needs of all individuals in the group, but lack of data or uncertainty in the data prevent being able to specify with confidence the percentage of individuals covered by this intake.

[a] As cholecalciferol. 1 μg cholecalciferol = 40 IU vitamin D.

[b] In the absence of adequate exposure to sunlight.

[c] As niacin equivalents (NE). 1 mg of niacin = 60 mg of tryptophan; 0-6 months = preformed niacin (not NE).

[d] As dietary folate equivalents (DFE). 1 DFE = 1 μg food folate = 0.6 μg of folic acid from fortified food or as a supplement taken on an empty stomach.

[e] Although AIs have been set for choline, there are few data to assess whether a dietary supply of choline is needed at all stages of the life cycle, and it may be that the choline requirement can be met by endogenous synthesis at some of these stages.

[g] In view of evidence linking folate intake with neural tube defects in the fetus, it is recommended that all women capable of becoming pregnant consume 400 μg from supplements or fortified foods in addition to intake of food folate from a varied diet.

[h] It is assumed that women will continue consuming 400 μg from supplements or fortified food until their pregnancy is confirmed and they enter prenatal care, which ordinarily occurs after the end of the periconceptional period—the critical time for formation of the neural tube.

Figure 7.7B

RECOMMENDED DIETARY ALLOWANCES TO APPLY PRECONCEPTIONALLY

FOOD AND NUTRITION BOARD, NATIONAL ACADEMY OF SCIENCES–NATIONAL RESEARCH COUNCIL
RECOMMENDED DIETARY ALLOWANCES,[a] Revised 1989 (Abridged)
Designed for the maintenance of good nutrition of practically all healthy people in the United States

Category	Protein (g)	Vitamin A (µg RE)[c]	Vitamin E (mg α-TE)[d]	Vitamin K (µg)	Vitamin C (mg)	Iron (mg)	Zinc (mg)	Iodine (µg)	Selenium (µg)
Pregnant	60	800	10	65	70	30	15	175	65

NOTE: This table does not include nutrients for which Dietary Reference Intakes have recently been established (see *Dietary Reference Intakes for Calcium, Phosphorus, Magnesium, Vitamin D, and Fluoride* [1997] and *Dietary Reference Intakes for Thiamin, Riboflavin, Niacin, Vitamin B₆, Folate, Vitamin B₁₂, Pantothenic Acid, Biotin, and Choline* [1998]).

[a] The allowances, expressed as average daily intakes over time, are intended to provide for individual variations among most normal persons as they live in the United States under usual environmental stresses. Diets should be based on a variety of common foods in order to provide other nutrients for which human requirements have been less well defined.

[c] Retinol equivalents. 1 retinol equivalent = 1 µg retinol or 6 µg β-carotene.

[d] α-Tocopherol equivalents. 1 mg d-α tocopherol = 1 α-TE.

strong determinant of hormonal levels because studies have shown that vegetarians have up to 20 percent lower estrogen levels than nonvegetarians of the same age.

Most vegetarians can actually be divided into three different dietary groups: lacto-ovovegetarians, who eat eggs, dairy products, and plants; lactovegetarians, who eat dairy products and plants; and vegans, who consume only plants. The vegans have the highest risk of problems due to their omission of meat, fish, eggs, and dairy products.

A major problem encountered by vegetarians as a group is protein deficiency. Proteins are made from amino acids. Of the 21 amino acids required by the human body, nine cannot be made in the body and must come from the diet. These nine critical amino acids (histidine, isoleucine, leucine, lysine, methionine, phenylalanine, threonine, tryptophan, and valine) are often called the "essential amino acids." Because plants usually only have a few of the essential amino acids required, vegetarians must make an effort to combine foods. They must take in *not only the 60 grams a day of protein required pre-conceptionally but, more importantly, a well-balanced variety of proteins*. Some foods that complement each other when combined to meet amino acid requirements are corn and black-eyed peas, beans and rice, and macaroni and cheese. Meeting the daily protein and amino acid requirement may be difficult for a strict vegetarian, but it can be accomplished if special attention is focused on consuming the right combinations of foods.

Zinc in the diet is usually supplied by animal products, so vegetarians can have a difficult time getting adequate amounts of this mineral. If you want to use vegetable sources of dietary zinc, some good sources are black-eyed peas, potatoes with the skin, green peas, and macaroni. As you can see from Figure 7.4, you'd have to eat a lot of black-eyed peas and potatoes to get the recommended daily allowance of 20 milligrams of zinc per day. A much simpler approach is to take a daily multivitamin.

Other common nutritional deficiencies in vegetarians include vitamin B_{12} and iron. For vegans, calcium and vitamin D deficiencies are also common. Vitamin B_{12} (also called riboflavin) is often deficient because plant foods don't contain this vitamin. Strict vegetarians must include fortified soy milk or a vitamin supplement in their diets to assure adequate amounts of vitamin B_{12}. Other sources of vitamin B_{12} include milk (and other dairy products), fortified breakfast cereals, and eggs.

It's clear that vegetarians are a high-risk group for preconceptional nutritional deficiencies. A limited number of vitamin and mineral deficiencies have been proven to delay conception, increase miscarriage rates, or result in birth defects; however, I suspect that future research will identify many more nutritional deficiencies with adverse reproductive consequences. Clearly, for most vegetarians the easiest and most reliable way to make sure you meet vitamin and mineral goals is to take a daily prenatal multivitamin tablet. If you choose to try to supplement all of the required nutrients through diet alone, it will be difficult but certainly possible.

NUTRITIONAL ALTERATIONS AS PREVENTION OR TREATMENT

Fibroids

If you remember from Chapter 2, fibroid tumors, also referred to as fibroids, uterine leiomyomata, or uterine myomas, are benign growths of smooth muscle tissue in the uterus. They are extremely common, affecting one in five Caucasian women

(20 percent) and up to one in three African-American women (33 percent). The influence of fibroids on fertility is controversial, but most experts agree that certain locations of fibroids—especially inside the uterine cavity or impinging on the uterine cavity—reduce fertility and increase miscarriage rates.

The role of diet in fibroid formation and treatment is poorly understood, but there appears to be a significant association between fibroids and what women eat. A research study by Dr. Francesca Chiaffarino and colleagues at the University of Milan, Italy, published in 1999, evaluated the diet of 843 women with fibroids compared to about 1,500 women without fibroids. Dr. Chiaffarino was able to show an association between beef and other red meats and the presence of fibroids. Green vegetables, and to a lesser extent fruits, seemed to protect against the formation of fibroids. This study also showed no association between fibroids and coffee, tea, or alcohol consumption. So just like your mother always told you—eat lots of fruits and vegetables!

Kue-chin-fu-ling-man (KBG) is a traditional Chinese herbal remedy that has been touted as a natural treatment for fibroids. Preliminary results have shown encouraging results in fibroid tumor shrinkage and symptomatic relief during menstrual periods. Like so many of the natural herbal therapies, little formal data exist to examine the efficacy of KBG in the treatment of fibroids. Additionally, due to the lack of testing it is uncertain whether this herbal treatment is safe around the time of conception. If you decide to try KBG for its potential therapeutic effects, I would suggest you use it only before or between attempts to become pregnant.

Vitamin E at 300 milligrams a day has also been used to treat uterine fibroids during pregnancy, beginning between week six and 12, but its effectiveness has not been established.

Endometriosis

To refresh your memory again from Chapter 2, endometriosis describes the presence of normal endometrial tissue (the uterine lining) outside of the uterus. Usually this tissue implants and grows in the pelvis, but in some cases it can be found outside the pelvic cavity. Endometriosis is common, affecting 2 to 5 percent of the female population. The associated inflammation in the pelvis often causes pain, and endometriosis is thought to decrease fertility by damaging the sperm and egg and interfering with fertilization. In more severe cases endometriosis can lead to scarring, reproductive organ damage, and eventually infertility.

The role of diet in the treatment or prevention of endometriosis is poorly understood. No well-designed research study has been performed to address the connection between diet and reproductive success in human patients with endometriosis. The limited data we have comes from animal experiments using fish oils that contain polyunsaturated fatty acids such as eicosapentaenoic acid (EPA) and docosahexaenoic acid (DHA). These kinds of fish oils, called omega-3 fatty acids, have received a lot of publicity in the recent past for promoting cardiovascular health.

The fatty acids EPA and DHA naturally inhibit the activity of an enzyme called cyclooxygenase. This enzyme produces other substances called prostaglandins, which play a key role in the inflammation associated with endometriosis. The idea is that EPA and DHA, by preventing the cyclooxygenase enzyme from making prostaglandins, can suppress this harmful inflammation and reduce the damage caused by endometriosis. At this point, certain animal experiments have suggested that dietary supplementation of EPA and DHA may achieve this effect. Whether this is true in humans is uncertain; we also don't know what the daily therapeutic dose would be.

Following the same line of reasoning, some authors have suggested avoiding foods with high amounts of certain prostaglandins, specifically arachidonic acid—a polyunsaturated fatty acid. Arachidonic acid naturally occurs in animal fat and liver. This means avoiding fatty meats, liver, and food products made from or with animal fat (such as pork rinds, lard, fatback, and anything cooked in grease).

Your own body also produces arachidonic acid from the linoleic acid you consume in your diet. Linoleic acid is a common and important unsaturated fatty acid found in many vegetable oils (such as sunflower, corn, safflower, soybean, cottonseed). If you wish to reduce linoleic acid in your diet, you can substitute olive oil for other vegetable oils, butter, or animal fats such as lard. There are no good studies to test the theory that reducing your intake of fatty meats, liver, animal fat, or linoleic acid will improve endometriosis. However, there could well be some benefit to these dietary changes. I wouldn't discourage anyone from trying this approach. Linoleic acid is an essential fatty acid (it is required for vital functions and your body cannot make it), so you wouldn't want to completely remove it from your diet.

If you have been diagnosed with endometriosis, it certainly wouldn't hurt to alter your diet for a few months and see if you note any improvement. EPA and DHA can also be purchased as nutritional supplements in tablet form. However, because of the uncertain amount of benefit, if you choose to try dietary therapy it should be combined with, not substituted for, proven medical treatments suggested by your physician.

NUTRITION AND MALE FERTILITY

Chapter 8 provides a detailed review of all of the key aspects a man should consider to maximize fertility. Here it should be noted that sperm counts and male reproductive function can suffer if men are significantly underweight, or have poor nutrition or an inadequate daily caloric intake. Deficiencies in zinc, selenium, and vitamins C, A, and E have also been implicated in decreased reproductive function. Some researchers have proposed a supplement of carnitine products, involved in fatty-acid metabolism, to improve sperm numbers and motility. In Chapter 8 I will provide details about the essential nutritional aspects of male fertility, and how to adjust your food and supplement intake accordingly.

Figure 7.8
FOOD PREPARATION ADVICE AND FOODS TO AVOID

- Produce—Wash all fruits and vegetables thoroughly to remove pesticide residues.
- Meat and Poultry—All meats should be cooked to well-done to decrease the chance of parasitic or bacterial contamination.
- Fish and Seafood—Sushi involves a small risk of a parasitic or bacterial contaminant, so you may choose to forgo this delicacy while trying to get pregnant and during the pregnancy. California rolls, made with cucumber and avocado, are vegetarian and may be a reasonable substitute. Additionally, consider sources of contamination if you are eating fish or seafood from small lakes, streams, or larger bodies of water. Swordfish may have higher levels of methylmercury, but an occasional serving of this fish shouldn't do any harm.

Figure 7.9
SUMMARY TABLE

Nutrition	1. Completely stop drinking caffeinated or alcoholic beverages.
	2. Do not take an aspirin a day to try to improve fertility.
	3. Take a prenatal vitamin daily beginning at least 30 days prior to conception.
	4. Consider additional iron supplementation if you have been previously diagnosed with iron-deficiency anemia.
	5. Assure dietary protein consumption of at least 60 to 75 grams per day.
	6. Vegetarians need to be especially vigilant about potential nutritional deficiencies.
	a. Protein intake usually must be increased. All nine essential amino acids need to be part of your diet.
	b. Common nutritional deficiencies in vegetarians, especially strict vegetarians (no eggs or milk), include lower levels of vitamin B_{12}, iron, calcium, and zinc.
	c. By taking a prenatal vitamin vegetarians can compensate for any vitamin and mineral deficiencies but not inadequate calcium or protein.
	7. If you have been diagnosed with fibroids, in addition to (not instead of) the recommendations made by your physician:
	a. Decrease consumption of red meat and other fatty meats and increase consumption of fruits and green vegetables.

Nutrition
 (continued)
	b. Consider taking 300 milligrams a day of vitamin E.
	
	 8. If you have been diagnosed with endometriosis, in addition to (not instead of) your doctor's recommendations:
	
	    a. Decrease intake of fatty meats, foods made with or of animal fat (for example, lard, bacon, pork rinds).
	
	    b. Switch cooking oil to olive oil and substitute olive oil for butter.
	
	    c. Increase intake of foods or take nutritional supplements containing omega-3 fatty acids (DHA and EPA), commonly found in fish.
	
	 9. If you have polycystic ovarian syndrome (PCOS):
	
	    a. Refer to the detailed review of PCOS and low-carbohydrate, high-protein diets in Chapter 6.
	
	 10. See Chapter 8 for male nutritional recommendations.

8

The Man's Role in Getting Pregnant Quickly

WHEN couples have difficulty getting pregnant, our society has a strong tendency to assume that the woman is responsible. As we noted earlier, male problems are the main cause of infertility in nearly 40 percent of cases, and 20 percent of the time it is a combination of male and female factors that lead to inability to conceive. This means that men and women are almost equally likely to contribute to fertility problems. Fertility should always be considered a couple's issue.

Internationally, it appears that sperm counts have decreased significantly during the last 40 to 50 years. The amount of the decrease is debated, but some studies estimate a reduction in sperm concentrations by as much as 50 percent since the 1940s and 1950s. Many scientists believe environmental toxins are responsible for this decrease. Various plastic and Styrofoam containers, skin creams, aerosol products, and many other items that we use daily have been found to contain estrogenlike compounds. In the modern world, these estrogenlike compounds are found everywhere around us; we cannot avoid them.

So far, the decrease in sperm counts does not seem to have significantly affected male fertility. This is probably because the average man has such a high concentration of sperm released during ejaculation that even a 50 percent reduction would not bring sperm counts down to critical levels. If the recent trend in sperm counts continues, some doctors estimate that a critical threshold in sperm numbers could eventually be reached, leading to a significant increase in male infertility.

There are many reasons why a man may have fertility problems. Anatomical abnormalities, medications, environmental toxins, underlying medical disorders, and social and psychological issues are the most common categories. Most of these problems have no symptoms, so the man usually has no suspicion that his fertility may be compromised. In this chapter, I will review the most common concerns and make specific recommendations. *Fortunately, simple changes in lifestyle and nutrition can often lead to significant improvements in male fertility.* I'll also talk about the common misconceptions regarding male fertility and the evidence for and against fertility-enhancing nutritional supplements.

Figure 8.1
RISK FACTORS FOR MALE INFERTILITY

- History of genital trauma or surgery
- Previous genital infection
- Lack of ejaculate during orgasm (retrograde ejaculation)
- Use of tobacco, alcohol, marijuana, cocaine
- Presence of a varicocele (dilated veins in the scrotum—often asymptomatic and unnoticed)
- Recent illness
- Chronic kidney or liver disease
- History of chemotherapy, or significant radiation to the genitals

- Age greater than 40
- Some medications (see Figure 8.3)
- Environmental toxins

ANATOMY

In Chapter 1 we reviewed the basic anatomy of the male reproductive system. In this chapter we will look at the most important aspects of male anatomy in more detail. The male reproductive system is designed to deposit a high concentration of good quality sperm close to the woman's cervix. Sperm production is quite sensitive to many external and internal influences, and this is where we'll focus our attention. The sperm are manufactured in the testicles. The testicles hang in the scrotum, a thin-walled sac, outside of the body. Muscles inside the scrotum contract and relax, raising and lowering the testicles.

The testicles are placed outside the body because the optimal temperature for sperm production is lower than 98.6 degrees Fahrenheit (37 degrees celsius), the body's normal core temperature. Many people have suspected that certain types of clothing or activities may lead to higher testicular temperatures and lower sperm production. Recent data indicates this concern has been overstated.

The prostate gland and the seminal vesicles secrete fluids for semen, the liquid ejaculated during orgasm. The prostate gland lies just below the base of the bladder and completely encircles the urethra. This is the tube that runs through the penis and carries urine from the bladder to the outside of the body. The prostate gland has ducts that empty into the urethra. The seminal vesicles are behind the prostate and secrete fluids into a tube called the vas deferens, which connects the

Figure 8.2

MALE REPRODUCTIVE ANATOMY

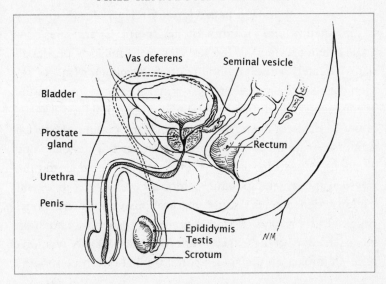

testicles to the urethra. Because the secretions from the prostate gland and seminal vesicles make up almost the entire volume of the semen, far more than sperm, the amount of semen ejaculated is not a good indicator of high or low sperm count. If a man doesn't ejaculate at all during an orgasm, he suffers from retrograde ejaculation and should see a physician.

The reproductive function of the penis is to be nothing more than a conduit to deposit the semen as close to the cervix as possible. Penile size has little effect on male fertility, because the average vaginal length is not longer than the average penis. When the male partner ejaculates, his semen flows into the urethra, and muscular contractions force the semen out the end of the penis. These rhythmic involuntary contractions create the sensation of orgasm for the male. Although male orgasm is necessary for pregnancy to occur, female orgasm is not.

SPERM

With few exceptions, a man's fertility relates almost entirely to the quality and quantity of his sperm. Sperm are constantly being formed in the testicles, with millions produced daily. Greater than 20 million sperm per milliliter (ml) of semen ejaculated is considered a normal sperm count, with the average sperm count around 60 million per milliliter. It takes about 74 days for a sperm to mature. Many common external influences can affect sperm production, such as tobacco and alcohol, viruses associated with the common cold or the flu, physical trauma, temperature, frequency of intercourse, nutritional deficiencies, some medications, and recreational drugs. The prolonged time required for sperm maturation means that any of these factors affecting male fertility wouldn't have an impact on the sperm count until about three months later.

Sperm have the best success at fertilizing the egg within two to three days of intercourse. The egg, however, can survive for no more than 12 to 24 hours (one day at most). Take these factors and combine them—the average woman has about 12 menstrual cycles per year, the egg only lives one day, and sperm perform best for two to three days—and you'll see there are only 36 days per year at most in which intercourse would be expected to have the highest chance of conception. This creates a narrow window of opportunity for the sperm and egg to unite.

The sperm can carry either an X chromosome or a Y chromosome. The chromosome in the sperm determines the sex of the offspring. All eggs bear an X chromosome, and depending on whether the sperm that fertilizes the egg contributes an X chromosome or a Y chromosome you have a boy (XY) or a girl (XX).

Whether an X-bearing sperm or a Y-bearing sperm reaches the egg first is totally random. Investigators have closely examined the differences between the X-bearing sperm and the Y-bearing sperm in order to find a practical way to allow couples to choose the sex of their child. Some investigators claim to have discovered effective ways to select the sex of a child by taking advantage of these differences. In Chapter 11 I will discuss common fallacies of sex selection as well as the few effective methods for choosing the sex of your baby.

Over-the-Counter Sperm Tests

Recently, commercially available home diagnostic screening tests for sperm counts have appeared in pharmacies. Baby Start Male Fertility Test (also called FertilMARQ) is the first FDA-approved test kit available to consumers. It allows you to test semen in the privacy of your own home. The test determines whether a man's sperm concentration (how many sperm per milliliter of semen) is above or below 20 million per milliliter. The test has an overall accuracy rate of 78 percent and it costs around $40.

The problem with this test is that there are three very important parts to a semen analysis, the sperm concentration, the swimming ability of the sperm (motility), and the appearance of the sperm (morphology). For example, if there are 50 million per milliliter of sperm but none of them are motile then this test would indicate the man is fertile. In reality he would be completely infertile.

I suggest that if you have reached the point that you are considering a semen analysis, just call your family practitioner or your wife's ob/gyn and they will be happy to order you a test at your local laboratory. The cost will be more, perhaps $75 to $150, but it will be well worth it.

ABSTINENCE PERIODS

A technician from a sperm bank told me that she had instructed a husband to "abstain for three days" prior to the day his sperm sample would be used to fertilize his wife's eggs in the laboratory. He expressed understanding and returned a week later to give the required sample. When asked when he had ejaculated last, he said he and his wife had intercourse that morning, "for good luck." The technician asked if he did not understand the instructions regarding "abstaining for three days" before providing a sample. He responded, "Oh, I thought you meant no beer."

It makes sense that having sex too frequently would result in decreased sperm counts; alternatively, a male could purposely abstain for a prolonged period to "save up" and increase his sperm counts. There is some truth to both these extremes if a man has sperm numbers that are at or below the lower limit of the normal range.

The recommended time interval to have intercourse is every 36 to 48 hours (one and a half to two days) during the most fertile period of the monthly cycle. Studies have shown that sex every day or more than once a day can lower sperm counts in some men, specifically those who have borderline sperm counts. If your sperm count is at the lower end of normal to begin with, then intercourse every day may decrease your fertility. For most couples having intercourse daily should not affect sperm counts, but the fact is that most men don't know their sperm counts, so the best suggestion is to have intercourse no more frequently than every 36 to 48 hours. Because sperm continue to fertilize an egg equally well for up to two to three days after ejaculation, intercourse every two days is frequent enough to always have viable sperm inside the female partner.

Most sperm banks ask sperm donors to be abstinent for at least two days but not more than five days before giving a sample. There is some research to show that abstaining for five to ten days might increase the count, but it probably doesn't significantly enhance fertility. Sperm age quickly, and after five to seven days some of the sperm begin to die. Although there are more sperm in the ejaculate of a man who abstains for more than a week, many of the older sperm cannot swim well anymore and do not contribute to fertility. *Abstaining for more than a few days—"saving up" for the time of ovulation—will not significantly increase your chances of getting pregnant quickly.*

NUTRITION

In earlier chapters, we reviewed the importance of nutrition for women in order for them to get pregnant quickly, reduce miscarriage risk, and decrease the risk of birth defects. Nutrition is a subject where the focus and attention has been directed almost solely on the female partner. In fact, optimizing nutrition in the male partner can be very important in getting pregnant as quickly as possible. Because sperm require 74 days to mature, *appropriate nutritional alterations need to be instituted about three months before trying to become pregnant if you want to get pregnant as quickly as possible.* This three-month rule will apply to many of the recommendations made in this chapter.

Antioxidants: Vitamins C and E

The words *antioxidant* and *free radical* are common terms these days, especially in skin care and nutritional-supplement advertising. Free radicals are chemicals containing oxygen in an unstable form. They can be formed in many ways, including through exposure to the sun and to certain chemicals, like those found in cigarettes.

Free radicals damage cells throughout the body. They cause

damage by changing normal cellular molecules into more free radicals, spreading through the cell in a domino effect. Among the parts of a cell damaged by free radicals is the DNA, which encodes the cell's vital genetic information. By interfering with the normal structure of the DNA, free radicals can kill the cells or cause mutations that alter the function of cells and may even lead to cancer.

Free oxygen radicals can be found in semen but are nearly absent in the semen of fertile men, whereas they are often found in high concentrations in the semen of infertile men. Some studies show that men with high levels of free radicals in their semen may have a seven times lower chance of conceiving than men with low levels of free radicals. The correlation between the high concentration of free oxygen radicals and decreased fertility indicates that sperm are being damaged by these chemicals.

The body has natural defenses against free radicals, but frequently they are not enough to counteract all the damage. Vitamins C and E are referred to as antioxidants because they neutralize the free oxygen radicals before they can damage cells. If taken separately, both vitamins C and E have been shown to decrease the amounts of the free oxygen radicals in semen. This suggests that taking more vitamins C and E may enhance your fertility. A study in 1996, by Dr. Eli Geva and colleagues at Tel Aviv University in Israel, showed that taking 300 milligrams of vitamin E twice a day improved fertilization rates for men with fertility problems. No similar study has been done for vitamin C.

Paradoxically, it turns out that taking vitamins C and E together may negate some of the benefits of each in reducing free oxygen radicals in the semen. Vitamin E appears to have a stronger relationship with improvement in semen quality; therefore, if you wish to take an antioxidant supplement *I would recommend taking 300 milligrams of vitamin E twice a day, but not supplementing vitamin C much more than the recommended daily allowance of 60 milligrams.* Perhaps increasing vitamin C to 250 milligrams is enough. This is not true for smokers, who should supplement vitamin C to more than 250 to 1,000 milligrams daily, because smoking can decrease the body's stores of vitamin C by up to one-half and chemicals in tobacco can lead to higher free-oxygen radicals in semen.

Selenium

Selenium is a mineral required by the body for many cellular functions and it also has antioxidant properties. Selenium deficiencies are correlated with an increased risk of male infertility. In 1998, Dr. R. Scott and colleagues from the Glasgow Royal Infirmary in Scotland published a study that evaluated selenium supplementation in Scottish males. That trial showed that selenium improved sperm quality in men who had low selenium levels before. *The study showed that the recommended daily allowance (RDA) of selenium is necessary for normal sperm production, but didn't indicate that selenium consumption over the RDA would lead to better sperm quality.*

Make sure you take the recommended daily allowance of selenium, but don't overload. Unlike the potential paradoxical relationship between vitamin C and vitamin E, selenium and vitamin E can be taken together. The easiest and most cost-effective way to assure meeting the RDA of selenium is to take a daily multivitamin that meets the RDA for all vitamins and minerals. Look at the bottle and it will tell you the percentage of RDA for each vitamin and mineral.

Other Vitamins and Minerals

Glutathione, zinc, and folate have also been shown to offer some benefit to male fertility. In general, meeting daily nutritional requirements is all that is necessary to maximize male fertility, and megadosing is not recommended. Remember that you can have too much of a good thing. I suggest a broad-spectrum multivitamin that meets the recommended dietary allowances. Most likely, we do not yet appreciate the relationship between male fertility and many other vitamins and minerals, so being certain that your multivitamin meets all of the RDAs is the best advice for now.

I should mention that taking a multivitamin each day does not obviate the need for good eating habits. A healthy well-balanced diet is vital to your general health. *A good diet, in addition to plenty of rest and exercise, will keep your immune system strong so that you don't get a viral or bacterial infection that could lower fertility for a certain time period.* You can obtain your necessary vitamins and minerals through a properly balanced diet, although the addition of a daily multivitamin assures meeting all requirements.

L-CARNITINE AND ACETYL L-CARNITINE

There are some nutritional supplements on the market that claim to improve male fertility. The latest and most talked-about are L-carnitine and acetyl L-carnitine, marketed together under the trade name of ProXeed (Sigma-Tau Pharmaceuticals; Gaithersburg, Maryland, *www.proxeed.com*). This is an over-the-counter dietary supplement that comes in a powder that is dissolved in liquid and taken twice a day. The manufacturer claims this supplement "promotes optimum sperm quality." The implication is that better-swimming sperm will result in more rapid conception.

L-carnitine and acetyl L-carnitine are water-soluble amines that occur naturally in the human body. These amines are normally made in the liver from amino acids and are involved in energy metabolism. L-carnitine and acetyl L-carnitine appear in much higher concentrations in the semen, and their exact role is uncertain. Studies have shown that the percentage of sperm that show motility, or swimming ability, is improved after taking L-carnitine and acetyl L-carnitine supplements for three to six months.

What I have been waiting for is research supporting the fact that this product actually helps couples get pregnant faster. Just because the sperm seem more motile when viewed under a microscope does not indicate that the couple will necessarily become pregnant faster. You can't assume that improved sperm motility equals better fertility or better health for your baby. My patience has paid off because in 2004 Dr. Giorgio Cavallini and colleagues published a study in the *Journal of Andrology* showing that L-carnitine (2 grams/day) + acetyl L-carnitine (1 gram/day) taken for six months significantly improved not only semen quality but also pregnancy rates. Pregnancy rates during the nine months of the study were 1.7 percent for the placebo group and 21.8 percent for the men taking the carnitines. Keep in mind this was a study of men with both low sperm concentrations and poor motility (swimming ability). There is no information I'm aware of to promote the use of carnitines in men in the general population, the majority of whom would be expected to have normal sperm counts.

ProXeed costs about $100 per month. You can purchase L-carnitine and acetyl L-carnitine separately as "generics" in health food stores. To match the dosage of ProXeed you need to take 1 gram (that's two 500-milligram tablets) of L-carnitine twice a day, and 500 milligrams of acetyl L-carnitine twice a day. More complete products that contain vitamins, minerals, and L-carnitine include Fertile One (*fertileone.com*—about

$90/month) and Conception XR (*www.conceptionxr.com*— about $90/month). FertileOne and Conception XR contain no acetyl L-carnitine, so you will need to supplement that separately.

EXERCISE

Excessive exercise does decrease fertility in some women. Men, however, do not have the same physiologic responses to exercise-related stress. Only a few studies have been performed to analyze the effect of exercise on male fertility. The results indicate that competitive athletes, in particular long-distance runners, can have mild decreases in their sperm counts. However, no cases have been found where infertility was specifically ascribed to a male partner's exercise habits. Men probably do not need to alter their exercise regimens when trying to get their partner pregnant.

SOCIAL HABITS AND RECREATIONAL DRUGS

Tobacco

Ironically, the most commonly encountered environmental toxins that negatively affect a man's fertility are ones to which men purposely expose themselves. Cigarettes have been shown to lower sperm counts and decrease sperm motility: smokers have fewer normal sperm, and the ones they have don't swim as well. In terms of getting pregnant as quickly as possible, men with borderline sperm numbers or quality may benefit from quitting smoking. Because few men know what their sperm counts are, I encourage all male partners to stop smoking as soon as possible in order to improve sperm quality. Remember, it takes about 74 days to produce sperm, so you should stop smoking at least three months prior to attempting to conceive in order to maximize your chances of conceiving a healthy baby rapidly.

Perhaps even more of a concern is that preconceptional *paternal* smoking has been associated with many problems you would never suspect, including an increased incidence of miscarriage, stillbirth, neural-tube defects, and some childhood cancers. At present, these are only noted associations and no cause-and-effect relationship has been established. Cigarettes contain many proven carcinogens (cancer-causing agents) and mutagens (agents that can cause mutations in the genetic code). In fact, there are over 2,500 chemicals found in tobacco smoke, and many of these have not been investigated for their effects on fertility or other health concerns.

Nicotine and many of the other chemicals found in cigarettes are concentrated in the semen so that their levels are actually higher in the semen than the blood. These chemicals may result in DNA damage and genetically defective sperm, resulting in potentially abnormal reproductive outcomes. A study by Dr. B. T. Ji and colleagues at Columbia University in 1997 published in the Journal of the *National Cancer Institute* showed that *preconceptional paternal smoking was associated with a 70 percent increase in the rate of childhood cancers*. Additional studies are needed, but given the serious nature of these associations, I strongly recommend against preconceptional paternal smoking.

Obstetricians have focused smoking cessation primarily on mothers, asking fathers only to avoid exposing their pregnant wife to secondhand smoke during the pregnancy. However, since preconceptional smoking by the male partner can decrease a couple's fertility and possibly increase the risk of abnormalities in the baby, the male partner should stop smoking before a couple tries to conceive.

After the baby is born you may want to resume smoking, but there will be new considerations. At your child's first office visit, the pediatrician will warn you that a smoking parent increases the child's risk of significant medical problems and even death. One of the strongest associations with Sudden Infant Death Syndrome (SIDS) is a parent who smokes.

Both the male and female partner must accept the fact that smoking will have to end with the decision to become pregnant. Studies have shown that if one partner tries to quit smoking while the other continues to smoke, the success rate is much lower than if both try to quit together. Many smoking-cessation products can be purchased over the counter. Most towns and cities have support groups for people trying to quit. Prescription medications also are available from your physician to help you stop smoking. It's a difficult thing to do, but the health benefits for you and your family are well worth it. *Remember, in order to derive maximum benefit from smoking cessation you should try to quit at least three months before conception.*

If you decide not to stop smoking prior to conception, make sure to have an adequate intake of vitamin C, as smoking can lower the body's levels of vitamin C by as much as one-half.

Alcohol and Caffeine

While female alcohol use can lead to a delay in conception, men appear to be able to drink alcohol in moderation without significantly affecting their sperm production and overall fertility. However, an association has been found between preconceptional alcohol use by the father and lower birthweight babies. There is still much we don't know about the relationship between preconceptional paternal alcohol use and fertility and health for the baby. *For this reason, I suggest that the man join his female partner in abstaining from alcohol for three months before attempting to conceive.*

Although men are less affected by moderate alcohol consumption than women, long-term excessive alcohol consumption by the man is a problem. It can decrease sperm production and sex drive and is suspected in causing an increased frequency of genetically defective sperm. There are no studies examining infrequent, short-term, excessive alcohol consumption, or binge drinking; however, it seems likely that sperm bathed in a high-alcohol environment could suffer damage. Once again, I recommend that alcohol consumption by the male partner be stopped or at least significantly curtailed well in advance of attempts at conception.

Little information is available on the relationship between caffeine and male fertility, but at present there seems to be little or no effect. We need good quality studies to be performed that will better examine this question.

Marijuana and Cocaine

Illicit drugs can have a substantial effect on male fertility. Marijuana is the most commonly used illicit drug in the United States. Around 20 million Americans smoke marijuana, and the vast majority are in their prime reproductive years. *Marijuana use can decrease testosterone (the major male hormone), resulting in lower sperm production, and may also cause a decreased sex drive.* Frequent users may have genetic damage to the chromosomes in their sperm. This raises the possibility of *a higher risk of miscarriage or birth defects.*

In 1992, Dr. William Hurd at the University of Michigan and colleagues showed that *cocaine also decreases sperm counts.*

For fast conception and a healthy baby, the male partner should avoid both marijuana and cocaine starting three months before trying to conceive. Also consider the bigger picture: Drug use may reveal that it is not the best time to start or expand a family.

Figure 8.3

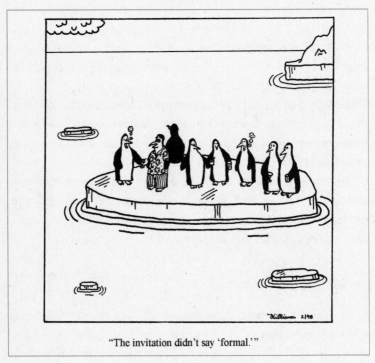

"The invitation didn't say 'formal.'"

MEDICATIONS

Some commonly used medications are often associated with erectile or ejaculatory dysfunction. Antihypertensives, anti-depressants, and many of the other classes of psychiatric medications are the most common offenders. A class of anti-hypertensives called calcium channel blockers may affect the ability of a man's sperm to fertilize the egg. The most common class of antidepressant medications, called the serotonin reuptake inhibitors (for example, Prozac and Zoloft), can leave men with an inability to achieve orgasm. Some men who take these medications must skip a dose or multiple doses prior to planned intercourse in order to be able to ejaculate. If you experience this side effect, you should have a discussion with your physician.

Some medications have anti–male hormone effects. A few of the most common medications that may suppress male hormones such as testosterone are spironolactone, a diuretic; ketoconazole, an antifungal; and cimetidine, an antacid/antiulcer medication. These medications can interfere with libido, or sex drive. Some steroidal medications, whether prescribed or illicit (such as the steroids used by bodybuilders), may also cause reproductive dysfunction. If you take any of these medications and experience side effects compromising your fertility or sex drive, you should discuss this with your physician. Frequently you can substitute these drugs with a different but equally effective medication.

Weight lifters, bodybuilders, football players, and other male athletes may sometimes take illicit anabolic steroids in order to build muscle. These men should realize that they risk testicular atrophy and poor sperm production, among other serious consequences. The steroid inhalers commonly used by asthmatics, on the other hand, should not cause a problem. Prescribed doses of oral steroids have the potential for decreasing fertility, but this depends on the dose and duration of treatment. *I always recommend discussing your medications with your physician before attempting to conceive. The vast majority of antifertility effects caused by drugs are temporary and can be relieved by either discontinuing the medication or switching to another medication with advice from your physician.*

Frequently associated with lower sperm counts are chemotherapy agents, used to treat cancer and some autoimmune disorders, and radiation when used for treatment. A man may suffer permanent loss of fertility after treatment with chemotherapy or radiation therapy. If faced with this situation, a man can protect his future reproductive options by providing and freezing sperm before he starts treatment. Fortunately, a simple chest X-ray or other routine diagnostic radiologic procedure should not cause any problems, especially if the testicles are shielded by a lead apron.

Figure 8.4
Drugs Associated with Decreased Male Fertility

- Antibiotics: sulfa drugs (a common component in many medications), nitrofurantoin (Macrobid, Macrodantin, Furadantin)
- Antidepressants
- Antihypertensives (many blood pressure medications)
- Antihormones: finasteride (Proscar, Propecia), flutamide (Eulexin), spironolactone (Aldactone)
- Alcohol
- Chemotherapy (cancer treatment)
- Cigarettes
- Cimetidine (Tagamet)
- Cocaine
- Diuretics (used to increase urine output to relieve swelling, treat hypertension, and some other purposes)
- Lipid-lowering agents (for cholesterol treatment)
- Narcotics
- Marijuana
- Some pesticides (dibromochloropropane)

STRESS

Both psychological and physical stress can contribute to a decrease in male fertility. The stress of a recent illness can temporarily lower sperm counts and/or sperm quality. This may be related to fever associated with the illness, or it may be the direct effect of a viral infection in the testicles. Psychological stress usually interferes with sex drive, erection, or ejaculation. There is also some data showing that stress and a negative self-image can adversely affect the percentage of normal sperm in the semen.

A study in 1999, by Dr. R. N. Clarke and colleagues from Brigham and Women's Hospital in Boston, evaluated the relationship between psychological stress and sperm quality in a group of 40 men undergoing in vitro fertilization (IVF) with their wives. According to this study, *increasing levels of stress led to a significant drop in sperm quality.*

Dealing with stress is a complicated issue, and many people find it difficult to learn how to cope effectively with stress. Your attitude is very important—to some extent we can choose to be positive or negative in our outlook on life. We can choose to deal with stress in different ways. Think about what things you do in order to cope with bad news, conflicts, excessive responsibilities, and other problems life brings to you. Each of us has developed our own coping mechanisms.

Most of these skills, whether good or bad, were learned from our parents while we were growing up. What did your parents do to deal with their stress? Was it effective or ineffective? Do you deal with stress in similar ways? Two of the most counterproductive coping mechanisms perpetuated in families are excessive alcohol use and the expression of excess anger or rage in the form of physical or verbal abuse to others.

Many people internalize the stress and make no attempt to

deal with it. Their coping mechanism is to act as if there is little or no stress around them. This is also ineffective. Unfortunately, people who handle stress in this way tend to deny that they are experiencing stress, and it can be particularly difficult to help them learn more effective ways to relieve the tension that daily life creates.

If you feel very stressed or tense in your daily life and you suspect that you're not handling this stress very well, consider trying out coping skills such as talking about the stressor with friends or family, exercising, reading, or practicing yoga. There are many books and programs available on handling stress effectively, as well as how-to books that devote themselves to one particular coping method.

It is important that you learn to recognize the stresses you are experiencing and then find constructive ways of dealing with them. For me one of the most effective ways to deal with stress is to talk it over with my wife. Another coping mechanism I frequently use is to go for a long run. It gives me a chance to think things through and gets rid of some of the aggression I may have built up. My wife likes to read to relax, whereas my mother will disappear into her garden after a difficult day. Each person has to discover what it is that clears the mind and reduces stress, and then find a way to do it when life becomes stressful. This will have a positive impact, not only on your fertility, but on your overall health and quality of life.

AGE

I remember watching an interview with Tony Randall and his wife, who was about 50 years his junior. They had recently had their first child together. The baby was happy and healthy, and you could tell that the interviewer just wanted to say, "Way to go, Tony!" In reality, there are far fewer reproductive problems associated with paternal age than with maternal age. Some evidence indicates that at the paternal age of 40, there may begin to be an increase in chromosomal mutations in sperm. This may slightly increase the chances for birth defects in the offspring. The increase in the risk of genetic problems with the sperm progresses slowly as men age. Men's decrease in fertility is also a very gradual process, and most men never reach a level where their fertility is compromised before they complete their family. Fortunately, in most cases the male partner does not have to experience the time pressures that are often a source of concern for women.

SEXUAL DYSFUNCTION

Sexual dysfunction is a broad term that includes all causes of problems with sexual function. Both psychological and medical problems can lead to abnormally low libido and erectile and ejaculatory dysfunction. Nearly all of these problems have effective treatments, although it may be necessary to consult a professional.

The most profound example of psychological sexual dysfunction I've ever seen involved a couple in which both partners thought that sexual intercourse was vulgar. Although they wanted children, neither one could bring themselves to have intercourse. The couple was referred to a clinical psychologist who evaluated them and decided they were quite normal, except for their aversion to sexual intercourse. They decided to have the husband provide a semen sample, which was then processed by our lab and injected into the wife's uterus using a technique called intrauterine insemination. They became pregnant on the first attempt.

Erectile dysfunction is not as uncommon as previously thought. It may be caused by a medical problem or a medication used to treat it, or by psychological issues. It's generally easy to determine whether erectile problems are due to psychological or physiological causes. All men have erections during rapid eye movement (REM) sleep and many wake up in the morning with an erection. If a man sees his erections are still occurring at night or when he awakens in the morning, he knows there is no physical impediment to becoming erect. Additionally, if the man cannot become erect with his partner but can masturbate successfully by himself, this also indicates a psychological cause. Whatever the reason for the erectile dysfunction, a visit to the family doctor or a urologist is always the first step.

Many men may find it difficult to perform on demand or if they are expected to have intercourse more frequently than every 24 to 36 hours, especially over a prolonged period of time. *Remember, you and your partner need not have intercourse any more frequently than every two days* up until the time of ovulation. This is frequent enough to maximize your chances of becoming pregnant as quickly as possible. Using a reliable method of ovulation prediction (see Chapter 5) will allow you to concentrate your intercourse only during the most fertile days of the menstrual cycle.

Despite having intercourse at the recommended times outlined in this book, it may happen that after a few months without success in getting pregnant, couples will start viewing these attempts as a frustrating monthly chore. Both partners may no longer see intercourse as exciting or fun. Extra encouragement and stimulation of the male partner may be needed to allow him to participate. Making sure that having intercourse always remains a romantic experience—with whatever serves to create a loving, intimate mood—will help ensure that both the man and woman fulfill their monthly "ob-ligations."

Libido, or sexual drive, is a complicated issue. There is more that is not known than is known about sex drive. Libido can be affected by medical problems and medications, but it is most commonly determined by psychological influences. Disturbances in sexual desire and sexual satisfaction are often interpersonal in origin. Couples often find that open communication and effective coping mechanisms for stress are the best ways to help libido problems. If you believe your sex drive has been significantly reduced due to psychological factors, you may want to consult a psychologist or psychiatrist who specializes in counseling for libido problems. On the other hand, if you note a change in sexual desire after instituting a medication, you should discuss this with your physician.

LUBRICANTS

Despite the indications on the lubricant packages, there is concern that even nonspermicidal lubricants have some spermicidal effects—meaning they kill sperm. The most natural way to get around the use of lubricants is to increase the amount of foreplay, which allows both the woman and the man to secrete natural lubricants. If that is not satisfactory, ordinary vegetable oil can be used safely.

BOXERS VS. BRIEFS—A HEATED DEBATE?

"Should I tell my husband that he needs to throw away his briefs in favor of boxer shorts?" This is a common question among couples, especially if they have not had success in rapidly conceiving. The idea is not as silly as it sounds. In fact, sperm are optimally produced when the testicles are kept cooler than the core body temperature. The theory is that tight-fitting briefs would hold the testicles too close to the body, leading to an elevated temperature and interfering with sperm production. Many physicians still hold this belief. During the time I was writing this book I was watching one of the national morning television shows, and I heard a "medical expert" recommend the use of boxers for this reason.

No one disputes the fact that significant prolonged elevations in testicular temperature can negatively affect sperm. The real question is not whether excessive heat can decrease fertility, but rather whether the subtle increases in testicular temperature caused by tight underwear result in impaired fertility. Is there any research available regarding this question? Would any respected medical investigator undertake such a study?

Two recent and well-designed studies offer the best data published to date on the influence of underwear type on male fertility. One study, by Dr. Christina Wang and colleagues from Harbor-University of California in 1997, had 21 male volunteers wear polyester-lined athletic supporters (jockstraps), some with aluminum lining, for one year. The scrotal temperatures increased on average by 1 degree Celsius, but there was no significant change in sperm counts. They concluded that briefs should not raise the temperature any more than polyester and aluminum-lined athletic supporters, therefore *briefs should not significantly affect sperm counts.*

The other study, by Drs. R. Munkelwitz and B. R. Gilbert from the State University of New York at Stony Brook, published in the *Journal of Urology* in 1998, evaluated the sperm numbers and quality of nearly 100 men. The men were categorized by "boxer" or "brief" groups, and semen analyses were obtained.

A portion of the men were switched to the alternative underwear type for comparison. The results showed that there were no significant differences in scrotal temperatures or sperm counts depending on underwear type. They also concluded that neither boxers nor briefs should affect fertility.

In a similar vein, there is a limited amount of research on the effect of hot tubs, hot baths, and saunas on sperm counts. A 1995 *New England Journal of Medicine* article by Dr. Stuart Howards at the University of Virginia indicated that excessive exposure to heat through the frequent use of saunas and hot tubs can result in decreased sperm counts. Whether this reduction in sperm numbers can delay conception in a couple probably relates to whether the man's sperm count was at the lower end of normal before the heat exposure. The average sperm count of men internationally is about 60 million per milliliter of semen. Because a normal sperm count is considered to be greater than 20 million per milliliter, most men have room for mild decreases in sperm numbers that might result from exposure to hot tubs, hot baths, or saunas. Most likely, sporadic use of saunas, hot tubs, and hot baths has little effect on the time to conception for most couples.

Some other causes of excess heat that may affect sperm counts include men with professions that require prolonged sitting or exposure to excessive heat. Truck drivers and taxi drivers, who are seated for very long periods of time, and welders are common examples. It seems reasonable to say that if young men who wore polyester- and aluminum-lined jockstraps didn't have significant changes in their sperm counts, then men who drive trucks, or sit for prolonged periods for other reasons, would have no significant decrease in their fertility either. Avid cyclists, whose testicles can suffer prolonged and potentially sperm-damaging pressures, can now buy a bicycle seat with the central portion removed to decrease the compression on the testicles.

CONCLUSION

Fertility is a couple's issue. Do not underestimate the importance of the male partner. There are many changes a man can make to maximize his fertility. Some of these alterations are simple, while others—such as quitting smoking—are quite difficult. Getting the appropriate nutrition, altering social habits, timing intercourse, forgoing lubricants, and attempting to modify life-stressors will maximize fertility in the male partner and contribute to a healthier baby.

Figure 8.5

*SUMMARY	
Social Habits	• Stop smoking and use of other tobacco products • Discontinue alcohol use (or significantly limit) • Discontinue marijuana and other illicit drugs • Avoid toxic environmental exposures
Nutrition	• 300mg vitamin E twice a day • L-carnitine 2 grams per day + acetyl-L-carnitine 1 gram per day (or order ProXeed)

SUMMARY (continued)	
	• If you smoke then take extra vitamin C—250 to 1,000 milligrams per day • Supplement with a daily multivitamin that includes the recommended dietary allowances of vitamins and minerals (avoid megadosing) • Additional selenium and folate may be required if a daily multivitamin has less than 100 percent of the recommended daily intake • If you want to be most complete order FertileOne or ConceptionXR but you will also need to supplement acetyl-L-carnitine 1 gram per day
Intercourse	• Intercourse every 36 to 48 hours beginning five days prior to anticipated ovulation. Combine timing of intercourse with a reliable method of ovulation prediction (see Chapter 5). • Do not use penile/vaginal lubricants. Increase foreplay or use vegetable oil.
"Heat"	• Wear any underwear you are most comfortable with (boxers or briefs) • Consider limiting the frequency of hot baths, hot tubs, saunas

	SUMMARY (continued)
Illnesses	• Get plenty of rest and a healthy diet for a strong immune system, to prevent illnesses which may temporarily decrease sperm counts
Exercise	• Unlike women, men do not appear to decrease their fertility with excessive exercise

*All recommendations should be instituted at least three months in advance of attempts to conceive for maximal benefit.

9

—

Sex and Fertility

AT last, we're getting to the most important part—making love! In previous chapters, we've spent a lot of time trying to optimize fertility in both the man and woman. At this point you and your partner should be ready to start trying to get pregnant. The question that this chapter will tackle is: What can you do in the bedroom to maximize your fertility?

I want to tell you up front that the topic of sex and fertility is filled with conjecture, and there is a paucity of reliable science to support most of the recommendations. If you "surf the Web" you will find all sorts of suggestions about sex to improve your chances of getting pregnant, including positions, timing, frequency of intercourse, maximizing sexual pleasure, and keeping the lights on, to name a few. What should you believe?

The most important recommendations regarding sexual intercourse and conception have already been reviewed in detail in Chapter 5. That chapter gave precise instructions on the appropriate timing of intercourse and predicting ovulation. Chapter 8 reviewed the optimal frequency of sexual intercourse, another aspect of sex that may enhance fertility in many couples.

The other influences on fertility to follow are certainly less important than timing of intercourse, but they may apply to you or your partner. For many couples, making love becomes a dreary monthly chore after a few months of trying to conceive without success. *By all means ignore the suggestions below, or suggestions from other sources, if they interfere with your pleasure or impair your sexual desire.* Every couple has their own unique sexual chemistry, and this is key to maintaining the excitement needed to make love regularly until conception occurs. This chapter will offer some insights about intercourse to help you maximize your chances of conceiving a healthy baby as quickly as possible while avoiding needless practices that may delay conception or inhibit your enjoyment.

NINE FERTILITY RECOMMENDATIONS TO USE IN THE BEDROOM

1. Positions for Sexual Intercourse

In general, the choice of sexual positions should have a limited effect on success rates; however, let's apply a little common sense to this issue. The exceptions would be if full penetration is not accessible with a certain position or if the semen is likely to run out of the vagina, such as when the woman is on top, standing, or bending over. It makes sense that after ejaculation the semen should stay in the vagina. For this reason, the classic "missionary" position would keep the semen at the level of the cervix, since the angle of the vagina naturally slopes downward when a woman lies on her back.

A good piece of advice for women, recommended by many infertility clinics, is to remain on your back after intercourse and have your partner place a pillow under your hips. This increases the downward angle of the vagina so that the semen pools up against your cervix. Stay in this position for at least 15 to 30 minutes. If it is nighttime, try to fall asleep on your back to keep the semen inside. Is there any research to prove this is helpful or not? No, but I warned you that this chapter would be short on data and long on common sense.

There is a commercially available product to promote the pooling of semen against the cervix. It is called Conception Curve (*www.conceptioncurve.com*—cost including S&H approximately $75). It is a wedge-shaped pillow that serves to raise the legs and hips following intercourse.

If you and your partner prefer a certain position and it helps sustain your sexual interest and pleasure, then don't let me talk you out of it. Back problems in men are extremely common, and many couples prefer to have the man "spoon up" behind the woman to take the stress off the man's back. Intercourse on your side keeps the vagina in a parallel position with the bed, so gravity shouldn't cause the semen to run out. For some obese couples, certain positions will allow penetration more effectively than others. Whatever the choice of position or reasoning behind it, I still recommend that the woman lie on her back and elevate her hips for a period of time after intercourse.

Chapter 11 reviews the most common recommendations regarding sexual positions and techniques for choosing the sex of your baby.

2. Lubricants

Many couples use lubricants to make sexual intercourse more enjoyable. Common brands of personal lubricants are K-Y Jelly (Advanced Care Products), Astroglide (Biofilm), Koromex PL (Quality Health), and Replens (Warner-Lambert).

Despite the indications on the packages, there is concern that even these nonspermicidal vaginal lubricants can kill sperm. The most physiological way to get around this drawback is to increase the amount of foreplay, allowing both the woman and the man to secrete natural lubricants. If that's not satisfactory, then vegetable oil can be used safely. Yes, you read it correctly—vegetable oil, bought at your neighborhood supermarket.

3. Desire, Arousal, and Satisfaction

Is satisfying intercourse important for fertility? No one disputes that mutually satisfying intercourse should be the goal for all couples, but when frequent intercourse is required to try to conceive, does a couple need to make every episode of sexual activity a chapter out of the *Kama Sutra*?

Many sources recommend that couples try to maximize sexual satisfaction when having intercourse in order to improve fertility. This includes prolonged foreplay and mutual orgasm. A few studies have examined these questions, and contrary to popular belief, optimizing fertility does not require maximal sexual pleasure or satisfaction for either partner.

The quality of the sperm sample produced by a man after extended sexual arousal and foreplay has been evaluated in a few studies. There was no difference in sperm quality or numbers between men who were highly sexually aroused before ejaculation and those who were not—although the men did note an improvement in ease of orgasm, intensity of orgasm, and overall satisfaction when they had prolonged stimulation prior to ejaculation.

The role of female orgasm in fertility is unclear. Besides the obvious sexual satisfaction it brings the woman, it may be that orgasm also functions to move the sperm into the uterus and up the Fallopian tubes. It is not known whether female orgasm improves fertility; however, many women who have never experienced orgasm have no problems with their fertility. It certainly doesn't hurt to achieve orgasm with each episode of intercourse, but it is probably not required to maximize fertility.

If conception takes several months to occur, many couples start to experience a decrease in their sex drive, also known as libido. Libido is a complicated issue with an enormous variety of contributing factors. Some couples initially do well, but later require extra stimulation of both partners. Also difficult for many men is the need to have intercourse on demand. If a couple is using an ovulation-prediction kit, the man has the added pressure of knowing that ovulation is occurring. For some men, this can lead to performance anxiety.

The use of "marital aids," such as erotic videos and magazines, is sometimes suggested to help with waning sexual desire and arousal. Extended foreplay can also improve the situation. As I mentioned earlier, each couple has a unique sexual chemistry. Over time partners learn what satisfies each other. Don't let this book or any other source push you into altering your normal intercourse in ways that make the experience less enjoyable or inhibit your libido.

4. Frequency of Intercourse for the Female Partner

We have reviewed optimal frequency of intercourse, or more accurately the frequency of ejaculation, to maximize fertility for the male partner. How about frequency of intercourse and its relationship to fertility in women? As it turns out, it appears that the fertility of a woman can change depending on how often she has intercourse.

A study by Dr. W. B. Cutler and colleagues at the Athena Institute for Women's Wellness Research compared the frequency of intercourse in young women with their basal-body-temperature (BBT) patterns. The BBT charts were used to indicate whether or not they ovulated each cycle. Women with regular sexual activity, at least weekly, had the highest incidence of fertile-type BBT charts, whereas sporadically sexually active women had a significantly lower proportion of apparently ovulatory cycles, and celibate women had the lowest incidence of fertile BBT charts. The study also found that self-stimulation to orgasm could not be substituted for actual intercourse to improve menstrual regularity. Although this study was small and had many limitations, it appears that frequent intercourse—at least once a week—in the months prior to conception may improve fertility by making the menstrual cycles more regular.

5. Oral Sex

Foreplay can involve any number of activities, and oral stimulation of either partner is common. There are some aspects of oral sex that could potentially impact on fertility. Enzymes present in the saliva and remaining on the penis when placed in the vagina could theoretically degrade the semen after ejaculation; however, the true effect of this would probably be minimal, and it is unlikely to affect fertility.

A few studies have attempted to evaluate whether oral sex could be a risk factor for decreased fertility. Sperm cells are foreign to a woman's body and are attacked by her immune system. The theory is that a woman who engages in oral intercourse and swallows her partner's semen could be sensitizing her body's immune system against that sperm. This could decrease fertility because the woman's body would start to manufacture antisperm antibodies. During normal vaginal intercourse the sperm would be attacked as a foreign cell by these anti-sperm antibodies, and the sperm wouldn't survive long enough to be able fertilize the egg. Interestingly, because sperm are unique to each man, antibodies made with previous partners should not affect other men's sperm.

The results of these studies have been mixed but it appears that oral intercourse is unlikely to be a significant risk factor for decreased fertility. As with many of the topics in this chapter, the results are not yet definitive. But if a couple enjoys oral stimulation and also wants to play it safe, then the woman should avoid ingesting the semen after ejaculation.

6. Douching

In numerous places in this book I have discouraged women from douching. Some authors, however, suggest that special douching can increase fertility. In addition, certain authors have offered specific douching recipes to influence the sex of the baby. Resist the urge to follow any of those recommendations. Do not try to mix up your own recipe of baking soda and water or vinegar in water douches to correct presumed vaginal pH problems or to try to improve the chances of choosing the sex of your baby. Douching will not improve your fertility and may lead to vaginal infection, which can ultimately affect your fertility (see Chapter 2).

7. Time of Day/Year

In 1894, Dr. Frederick A. Cook traveled to Greenland and made some interesting observations about the native inhabitants. Dr. Cook noted that during the four-month Arctic winter, when it stayed dark constantly, "not more than one woman in ten [were] menstruating." The brain is able to follow patterns of daytime and nighttime, and it keeps track of the length of daylight during the four seasons. All animals exhibit patterns of hormonal release correlated with the environment; these are called circadian rhythms. External influences such as length of day, temperature, diet, and activity can influence these rhythms.

You become more aware of your circadian rhythms when you experience jet lag. We have all felt the undeniable effects of crossing time zones, and the need for about one day per time zone to reestablish appropriate synchronization. Recently, "light therapy" has been proposed for travelers to help them adjust more rapidly to time changes.

Recent advances in our understanding of anatomy and physiology have given some indication of the possible connections between circadian rhythms and fertility. The pineal gland, or pineal body, is a part of the brain that closely monitors periods of light and dark and secretes a hormone called melatonin in response to these patterns. In animal experiments, the pineal gland has been shown to have an important role in reproduction. Soltriol, a form of vitamin D, is a hormone that is produced in response to sunlight, and some researchers believe it influences the centers of the brain that control reproduction. Melatonin, soltriol, and some other light-sensitive hormones are known to influence the reproductive system; however, these relationships are poorly understood.

Some researchers have proposed "light therapy" to improve fertility, but no exact regimen has been demonstrated. Frequent exposure to a limited amount of sunlight is probably healthy and fertility enhancing. Certainly regular activity or relaxation outdoors in the sunlight would be expected to promote fertility, both through the production of the light-sensitive hormones and through stress reduction.

Having intercourse at a certain time of day appears to be less important. Some sources suggest making love with the lights on or during the daytime because light promotes fertility, but this is unproven. As I said before, nighttime intercourse is often more advantageous, because the woman can go to sleep on her back allowing the semen to pool against the cervix for a prolonged period of time. In theory at least, this would increase the number of sperm entering the female reproductive tract and should raise the chances that a sperm will find the egg.

Conception rates do fluctuate throughout the year. But, overall, this has little applicability, because the differences between seasons are not substantial enough to encourage you to alter your pregnancy timetable.

8. Extracurricular Ejaculations

A piece of practical advice addresses masturbation. Chapter 8 reviewed the optimal frequency of sexual intercourse in terms of sperm counts. I suggested that a couple space their intercourse every 36 to 48 hours during the most fertile period, in order to maximize sperm counts. The majority of men have normal sperm counts and more frequent intercourse probably won't affect fertility. Because men don't know their sperm counts, and intercourse every 48 hours has been shown to be equally effective for conception as daily intercourse, I recommend that couples space out their intercourse to every 36 to 48 hours during the most fertile time of the menstrual cycle until a reliable ovulation-prediction method indicates when ovulation will occur.

Studies indicate that the majority of men masturbate, so it's not unlikely the male partner is actually ejaculating more often than the frequency of intercourse with his partner. Every two days may not be frequent enough for some men. However, as I noted above, additional ejaculations between intercourse could contribute to less than optimal semen samples in men who have sperm numbers in the lower end of the normal range.

9. Electric Blankets/Waterbeds

Some researchers have raised the issue of an increased risk for miscarriage, birth defects, and decreased fertility from the electromagnetic fields generated by electric blankets or the heating mechanisms of waterbeds. There have been a few studies designed to evaluate this question. The results have revealed slightly higher rates of miscarriage and decreased fertility in users of these products; however, the studies were not definitive.

Electromagnetic measurements indicate that the exposure from electric blankets is more than twice as high as that from the heating units of waterbeds. Hopefully, a definitive answer regarding electromagnetic exposure and fertility or miscarriage will come from the California Pregnancy Outcome Study, a component of which is evaluating that kind of association. Although I doubt there's a strong relationship between these products and poor reproductive outcomes, my recommendation for you and your partner is to replace your electric blankets with a couple of regular blankets or a comforter while you are trying to conceive and during your pregnancy. At this point in time, I don't think it is necessary to buy a new bed to replace your waterbed, since the electromagnetic fields generated by waterbeds appear to be significantly lower than those from electric blankets.

CONCLUSIONS

The recommendations above will apply to many readers, and I hope they help. A lot of what I have told you involves common sense because there is little data available to definitively answer many of the questions raised in this chapter. Some things to keep in mind are the increased risk of harmful reproductive consequences from douching, the likely spermicidal effects of lubricant use, the possible connections between reduced fertility and electric blankets, the potential importance of sun exposure, and the fertility-enhancing results of frequent intercourse for the woman. Couples should benefit from having the woman lie on her back and elevate her hips for at least 15 to 30 minutes after intercourse. Once again, the most important recommendations to take away from this chapter are— don't take things too seriously, don't alter your sexual habits if this reduces your pleasure or motivation, and most of all, enjoy yourselves!

10

—

Turning Back the Clock:
Getting Pregnant at 35 and Older

THE last few decades have seen rapidly changing patterns in childbearing. One in five women now wait until they are 35 years old or older before having children. In the United States, between 1988 and 1998, the number of women over 40 having babies more than doubled, increasing from about 41,000 to nearly 85,000. This shift in the timing of pregnancies has been due mainly to women's desire to reach a higher level of education, establish themselves in their careers, and achieve financial stability before starting their families. Remarriage has also been a key factor contributing to the number of pregnancies in women 35 years of age and older.

The issues associated with a delay in childbearing have brought significant anxiety, even alarm, for many women. If you are one of these women, let me reassure you that *for the vast majority of those who elect to delay childbearing until they have fulfilled other important life goals, everything will work out fine.*

Unfortunately, the mass media has overdramatized the situation, making many people believe that getting pregnant over age 30 will be difficult and pregnancies over age 35 will be fraught with medical complications and birth defects. This is just not true. The odds of getting pregnant in a reasonable time frame and delivering a healthy baby are in your favor at any age until about age forty. Of course, younger is better in terms of reproduction so don't try to break the existing record (according to the *Guinness Book of World Records*) for the oldest spontaneous (unassisted by technology) pregnancy in a woman at 57 years and 120 days old. It is true that delayed childbearing increases the risk of adverse fertility and pregnancy consequences and the need for physician assistance in order to conceive, and this chapter will review those risks in detail.

I am frequently asked by patients how much they should be concerned about their age. I tell these patients to think of age and fertility as a continuum. Fertility is highest around 20 years old and then declines gradually until the late thirties. There is no dramatic change in the rate of decline until the late thirties. The difference between 29 years old and 30 years old, or 34 years old and 35 years old, is negligible. Once women have entered their late thirties, the rate of decline in fertility becomes more dramatic, and by the mid-forties pregnancies that progress to delivery are uncommon. Not only does conception become difficult for this age group, but the rate of miscarriage also goes up. That being said, there is a lot of variability. Some 41-year-old women have the fertility of a 35-year-old—and vice versa.

The average age of menopause is 51 years. This means that a significant number of normal women will go through menopause in their mid-forties, while others will wait until their mid-fifties. Smoking cigarettes and alcohol consumption have been consistently demonstrated to be associated with an early natural menopause. Stopping these habits may delay the onset of your menopause. A study by Dr. David Torgerson and colleagues from the University of York in the United Kingdom in 1997 showed that the risk was six times higher for a woman to have an early menopause (at less than 45 years) if her mother experienced an early menopause. Finding out the age of menopause for other women in your family should help you predict when yours will occur. This can be especially important for those families with a history of earlier menopause. Also remember that menopause does not occur all of a sudden. Ten years or more prior to menopause the ovaries slowly start to fail; this is what reproductive specialists call "a loss of ovarian reserve."

When couples delay childbearing, they often feel more pressure to conceive quickly because they have less time to complete their family before their fertility and reproductive outcomes are jeopardized. If you are in this position, you may feel extra anxiety around the issue of conception. However, keep in mind that although it may take a woman longer to become pregnant in her late thirties, the chances are very good that she will succeed in having the healthy baby she desires.

Jill, 38, exemplified another concern shared by many professional women who postpone their childbearing: not only did she want to conceive quickly, but she also wanted it to occur during one specific month in order to time her delivery around the completion of a project for work. When professional women defer starting a family, they have often risen in the ranks of their profession to a level where their business responsibilities need to be factored in with their own personal schedules. In my practice I have a lot of patients from the University of Virginia. I commonly see faculty and graduate students who seek my advice on getting pregnant during the months of September or October. Couples on an academic calendar naturally want to try to conceive nine months before the end of the school year, so they can have the summer to be with their new baby.

No one can turn back the clock, but if you apply the simple interventions found in this book regarding preconceptional care, pre-pregnancy nutrition, ovulation prediction, social habits, the male partner, and many other issues, you will get pregnant faster and improve your chances up front of having a healthy baby. Women in this age category should be especially diligent about following preconceptional recommendations, because they are more likely to experience reproductive problems and have less time available to correct them.

HOW AND WHY FERTILITY CHANGES WITH AGE

Ovarian Changes

Of course, there is such a thing as a "biological clock." If a woman is otherwise healthy, the most important factor determining her fertility is her age. Women become less fertile mainly due to the aging of the ovaries. At puberty the ovaries contain about 400,000 eggs. As women age so do the ovaries and the eggs that remain inside. With each monthly ovulation a group, or cohort, of eggs (estimated at as many as 500 to 1,000) is recruited, but only a single egg enters the Fallopian tubes (unless the woman has a predisposition to fraternal twins). The remaining eggs are reabsorbed by the ovaries and lost.

By the time of menopause no eggs remain, but fertility is significantly reduced for up to a decade prior to menopause as ovarian function wanes. One explanation for this reduction in fertility is that the body may choose the most responsive and highest quality eggs first, so by the late thirties and early forties only the poorer quality eggs remain—not poorer quality in terms of the babies produced, but in regard to how easily conception occurs and how high the risk of miscarriage and chromosomal problems becomes. The other theory is that the eggs, like all the other cells in the body, simply decline in function over time. Whatever the cause, the quality of the eggs diminishes parallel to the decline in fertility. The eggs become more difficult to fertilize, and when they do become embryos there is a higher risk of miscarriage. With increasing age there is also a gradual increase in the rate of chromosomal abnormalities, which is chiefly responsible for the increased risk of miscarriage. Therefore, older women experience two sources of concern: delayed conception and a higher rate of miscarriage.

Figure 10.1

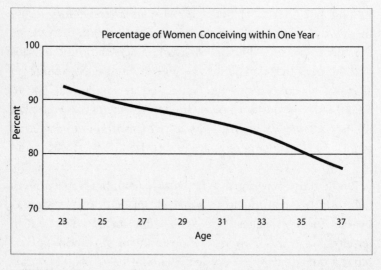

Adapted with permission of the Alan Guttmacher Institute from J. Bongaarts, "Infertility After Age 30: A False Alarm." *Family Planning Perspectives*, vol. 14, no. 2 (1982): 77.

Chromosome Problems and Age

Lynda, 34, came to see me because she was concerned about Down's syndrome. She said, "My husband and I really want to get pregnant this year before all of the increased risks of Down's syndrome and other genetic problems start when I turn 35." When I told her that most Down's syndrome babies are born to women younger than she, Lynda was shocked. Of course, there are many more pregnancies in younger women overall; therefore, despite the higher risk for chromosomal abnormalities in older mothers, most Down's syndrome babies have young mothers. Like infertility, the risk of genetic abnormalities slowly increases as women age. There is no magic to age 35.

With rare exceptions, every cell in the body has chromosomes. These chromosomes contain the genetic code that makes us who we are. (See Chapter 3 for more details on our chromosomes and DNA.) During the union of sperm and egg, chromosomes or segments of chromosomes may be lost, or too many chromosomes or segments may be retained in an embryo. These situations can result in functional abnormalities in the offspring.

The most well-known example is Down's syndrome, also known as Trisomy 21. In a Down's syndrome baby, the cells contain three copies of the twenty-first chromosome, which is one too many chromosomes. This leads to mental retardation and other problems including characteristic facial features, short stature, and heart defects. Other common chromosomal abnormalities that increase with age are Trisomy 18, 13, and 16. In fact, most chromosomal abnormalities cause such severe abnormalities in the affected fetuses that early miscarriage occurs. It is the rare chromosomally abnormal baby that is live born.

The increase in chromosomally abnormal children follows a gradual upward curve similar to the reduction in fertility with age. As I indicated earlier, more children with chromosomal problems are born to young mothers (younger than 35) than to older ones simply because there are more younger mothers than older ones. However, screening for abnormal chromosomes in the fetus isn't usually performed during pregnancy until the woman is 35 years old. This is because the screening itself, performed either by chorionic villus sampling (CVS) or amniocentesis during the early second trimester, involves a risk of miscarriage in about one in 200 procedures. The one-in-200 chance of miscarriage is equivalent to the risk of a 35-year-old woman having a baby with a chromosomal abnormality. Because women under 35 (with no risk factors) have a lower than one-in-200 chance of having a baby with a chromosomal problem, they'd actually be at higher risk of complications just by taking the test. That is why 35 years has become the official age physicians begin offering genetic screening to women. Keep in mind that this one-in-200 chance of abnormalities is really only 0.5 percent, so *even a woman of 35 still has a 99.5 percent chance that the chromosomes are normal.*

Amniocentesis is the most common approach to chromosome testing of a fetus and is usually performed between 16 and 18 weeks into the pregnancy. In this procedure, a doctor places a needle through the mother's abdomen into the sac of amniotic fluid, using ultrasound guidance to avoid the baby, and removes a few ounces of the fluid to be tested in a genetics laboratory. The fluid contains enough cells to reveal the karyotype, or chromosome analysis, of the baby.

Maternal age is by far the most important risk factor for chromosomal abnormalities, but the father's age is also associated with a higher risk. Paternal age can cause an increased incidence of trisomies, such as Down's syndrome, and gene mutations

Figure 10.2

INCREASED RISK OF A CHROMOSOME
ANOMALY WITH AGE

Maternal Age (years)	Risk for Down Syndrome	Total Risk for Chromosomal Abnormalities
20	1/1,667	1/526
25	1/1,250	1/476
30	1/952	1/385
35	1/378	1/192
40	1/106	1/66
41	1/82	1/53
42	1/63	1/42
43	1/49	1/33
44	1/38	1/26
45	1/30	1/21
46	1/23	1/16
47	1/18	1/13
48	1/14	1/10
49	1/11	1/8

This table originally appeared in Creasy and Resnick, eds. *Maternal Fetal Medicine: Practice and Principles.* (Philadelphia: W. B. Saunders, 1994), 71. Reproduced with permission from the publisher, Harcourt Health Sciences.

resulting in various genetic diseases. The increase in paternal risk appears to begin at age 40, but compared to the maternal influence the risks contributed by an older father are small.

WHAT CAN BE DONE TO REDUCE YOUR CHANCES OF A CHROMOSOME PROBLEM, BIRTH DEFECT, OR MISCARRIAGE?

There is no way you can turn back time; however, some of the other contributing factors to chromosome problems, reduced fertility, and miscarriage *can* be altered. Social habits, nutrition, and environmental toxins can all increase the risk of these adverse outcomes.

A good example is when the father smokes prior to conception. In Chapter 8 I reviewed the recent research indicating that preconceptional *paternal* smoking has been associated with many problems you would never suspect, including an increased incidence of miscarriage, stillbirth, neural-tube defects, and some childhood cancers. If the father stops smoking at least three months before conception, it may reduce the overall risk of reproductive problems regardless of the mother's age.

Eggs are not constantly produced throughout one's lifetime like sperm. In spite of this, it appears that some preconceptional maternal behaviors, such as poor nutrition, smoking, and alcohol use/abuse, may lead to a higher risk of chromosomal abnormalities in the offspring and these factors could increase the risk of birth defects, miscarriage, and a difficult pregnancy. Therefore, *it's especially important that women 35*

Figure 10.3

Risk of Miscarriage with Increased Age

Maternal Age (Years)	Spontaneous Abortion(%)
15-19	9.9
20-24	9.5
25-29	10
30-34	11.7
35-39	17.7
40-44	33.8
≥45	53.2

From P.R. Gindoff and R. Jewelewicz. "Reproductive Potential in the Older Woman." *Fertility and Sterility*, 46 (1986): 989. With permission from the American Society for Reproductive Medicine and Elsevier Science, copyright © 1986.

or older eat well, get ample vitamins, minerals, and protein, and stop smoking and drinking alcohol and caffeine-containing products when they are trying to become pregnant and during the pregnancy.

Poor maternal control of diabetes prior to conception does not increase the risk of chromosomal abnormalities in the fetus, but it does dramatically increase the chance of birth defects. Heart, brain, spinal cord, lower limb, and kidney defects are the most common. When a diabetic woman adequately controls her sugars before conceiving, her risk of birth defects is nearly the same as nondiabetic mothers. Keep in mind that *older mothers have an increased risk of being diabetic because the incidence of diabetes increases with age.* If you have a family history of diabetes, suspect you may have polycystic ovarian syndrome or diabetes, or are significantly overweight, I suggest you see your family doctor or obstetrician/gynecologist and have a screening test for diabetes prior to conception.

MISCARRIAGE RISK AND AGE

The risk of miscarriage dramatically increases with age. By age 45, over 50 percent of all pregnancies will end in miscarriage. This compares to about a 10 percent chance of miscarriage in a 20-year-old (see Figure 10.3). Because this risk can be elevated by many different factors, women 35 years and older will want to make sure they have optimally lowered their other risk factors for miscarriage, including *bacterial vaginosis* (Chapter 2), *fibroids* (Chapter 2), *weight and exercise* (Chapter 6), *caffeine and tobacco use* (Chapters 3 and 8), *environmental toxins* (Chapter 3), *medications and some chronic medical problems* (Chapter 3), and *nutrition* (Chapters 3 and 7). In general, these are the same factors that influence general fertility and birth defects.

MEDICAL PROBLEMS

The older you become, the more likely it is that you or your partner will have acquired a medical problem. Nearly all groups of medical disorders and gynecological problems increase in frequency with age. Some of these medical problems are easily preventable, but even when a couple cannot avoid a fertility-impairing medical disorder they can usually take steps to enhance their chances of having a healthy baby in a reasonable time frame.

An example of a male disorder that becomes more frequent with age is varicoceles, or swollen veins around the testicles. Varicoceles are often asymptomatic but can decrease sperm counts and sperm quality. In fact, most men with low sperm counts have no symptoms, and poor semen quality is the last thing they expect.

Common gynecological problems that are seen more frequently in older women and have a potential impact on fertility include endometriosis, previous pelvic infection, fibroids in the uterus, polycystic ovarian syndrome or irregular menstrual cycles from any cause, and a history of previous pelvic surgery. In Chapter 2 I reviewed these common problems and made an effort to reassure women that these problems usually don't interfere with timely conception. Even if you have or had one or more of these gynecological problems, the odds are still in your favor. In Chapter 2 and many subsequent chapters I have specifically reviewed prevention and treatment strategies for women with these problems.

Nongynecologic medical problems (such as adult-onset diabetes mellitus or hypertension) and associated medications used to treat the disorders can sometimes interfere with fertility and increase the risk for pregnancy complications. Chapter 3 reviewed many of the nongynecologic medical problems and medications used to treat them. If you have any chronic medical problem, you should discuss it with your obstetrician/gynecologist or family doctor *before* becoming pregnant.

MATERNAL PREGNANCY RISKS AT AGE 35 OR OLDER

Although this book focuses on preconceptional concerns, I want to mention the relationship between maternal age and pregnancy complications. Because older women have had more time to acquire medical problems, older mothers are more likely to have health complications during pregnancy. If you have a chronic medical problem, such as hypertension, you should contact your obstetrician/gynecologist or family practitioner about the influence the disorder may have on conception and pregnancy, as well as how pregnancy might affect the medical disorder (that is, will pregnancy worsen it or improve it). Also, your doctor may want to change your medication(s) if there is an alternative that would be safer during conception and pregnancy.

Delayed childbearing has been associated with an increased risk of maternal problems; however, the good news is that *with good preconceptional and prenatal care, outcomes can approach those of younger pregnancies.* Keep in mind that even without preexisting medical problems such as diabetes or hypertension, older women are more likely to develop these during pregnancy. Sometimes your doctor will want to refer you to a perinatologist, also called a maternal-fetal medicine or high-risk pregnancy specialist, to assess any medical problems or risk factors. As I mentioned above, always find out if it is safe to become pregnant while taking a certain medication. If your medication isn't safe during pregnancy, a different medication can often be substituted during the time you are trying to conceive and during the pregnancy. Remember, *many of the medications that are toxic to early pregnancies can cause malformations before women even know they are pregnant.*

For the reasons noted above and some unknown contributing factors, women over 40 are at higher risk for difficult deliveries. Dr. William Gilbert, from the University of California, Davis, published a study in 1999 of more than 24,000 women age 40 and older, which showed that almost 50 percent of the women in this group required a cesarean section for delivery. In addition, the rates of birth asphyxia, poor fetal growth, abnormal positions of the baby in the womb, and gestational diabetes were significantly higher. Despite these data, Dr. Gilbert was quoted by NBC news as saying, "The good news is that from our study, we found that the vast majority of women who become pregnant in their forties have a wonderful outcome." Therefore, although women in this age group have to keep a careful watch on the course of the pregnancy, it is appropriate to be optimistic.

HOW LONG SHOULD IT TAKE TO GET PREGNANT?

Overall, 85 to 90 percent of couples will become pregnant after trying to conceive for one year. This statistic is an average and includes data from couples of all ages. It would be most accurate for couples at approximately age 30. At age 20 a couple has a 93 percent chance of getting pregnant without any trouble within a 12-month period. By age 40, the chance of conceiving within one year is about 70 percent. Once a woman reaches the age of 45 pregnancy is uncommon. This doesn't take into consideration the fact that the rate of miscarriage is much higher in a 40-year-old woman than a 20-year-old woman. However, the 70 percent statistic means that *even at the age of 40, the odds of conceiving in a reasonable amount of time are more than twice as high as the chances of a problem in becoming pregnant.*

Another way to evaluate the decline in fertility with age is to look at the probability of becoming pregnant each month if intercourse is timed appropriately. A 20-year-old couple has about a 25 to 30 percent chance of becoming pregnant each month. In contrast, the likelihood of conceiving each month for a 40-year-old couple is no better than 10 to 15 percent. By the middle forties the chances of becoming pregnant each month are estimated to be less than 5 percent, and greater than 90 percent of 45-year-old women will not become pregnant by the end of one year of attempts.

The data underlying these numbers come from the years before good quality home ovulation-prediction kits, preconceptional care, and other important resources that are easily accessible today. Most likely, with modern information and technology the rate of conception each month could be higher at nearly all ages. Nevertheless, you should hold a realistic expectation of the time it may take to become pregnant, based on your age.

WHEN SHOULD YOU GET FERTILITY TESTING BEFORE ATTEMPTING TO CONCEIVE?

In general, unless you have a specific problem or medical history that would be expected to interfere with your chances of conceiving (such as irregular or absent menstrual cycles), you should try to conceive on your own before considering specific diagnostic fertility testing. Of course there are exceptions, and the older couple is one of them. Although I recommend a preconceptional check-up for all couples regardless of age, I *strongly encourage* a doctor's visit for couples 35 years and older. In addition to following all the preconceptional recommendations outlined in Chapter 3, couples in their late thirties or older may want to specifically consider preconceptional screening for ovarian function and sperm quality.

By far the easiest and most cost-effective screening test for older couples who are planning to start trying to conceive is a semen analysis. It is a relatively cheap test (about $75 to $150) and involves no risk. Because as many as 40 percent of infertile couples are infertile because of the man, we shouldn't forget him. Especially if the female partner is age 40 or older, a screening test of the semen quality may help to prevent a significant delay in conception.

We have mentioned follicle stimulating hormone (FSH) and luteinizing hormone (LH) many times throughout the book already. These hormones, released by the brain, are responsible for stimulating the ovary to produce a mature egg and to release it in the process of ovulation. The aging ovaries become progressively less responsive to these hormones. As the ovaries lose their sensitivity to FSH, the brain releases more and more of this hormone in an attempt to aggressively stimulate the unresponsive ovaries. The resulting rise in FSH levels serves as a good marker for poor ovarian function, also called "diminished ovarian reserve."

For women in their late thirties who are planning to try to conceive, but most useful in women 40 years or older, a simple blood test can screen for FSH and estradiol (a type of estrogen) to determine if the ovaries have diminished reserve. Women in this age group can ask their physician about this test before trying to get pregnant. In Chapter 12 I go into detail about FSH testing and other ways of assessing ovarian function. I merely want to introduce these screening tests to you here.

The basic FSH screening test is administered on the third day of the menstrual cycle. A high FSH value alone or combined with an elevated estradiol level indicates that your chances of conceiving are significantly compromised. The level of FSH used as a cutoff for abnormal depends on the laboratory, your age, and your clinical history and must be interpreted by your doctor.

A more sensitive test of ovarian function is called the clomiphene citrate challenge test (CCCT). This test is more complicated—it involves two separate blood draws and an oral ovulation-inducing medication called clomiphene citrate administered for five days at the beginning of your menstrual cycle. Your obstetrician/gynecologist may need to consult with a reproductive endocrinologist because there are subtleties to interpreting the results of this test and it is probably a test that may not be commonly ordered by your obstetrician/gynecologist or family practitioner. The alternative is to have your preconceptional visit with a reproductive endocrinologist in your community. Your doctor may offer you the CCCT instead of or in addition to the FSH and estradiol test, which is given on day number 3 of your cycle, and you can discuss during your preconceptional office visit which of the two tests to perform. Keep in mind that a normal result from either of these screening tests merely indicates that your ovarian function is not poorer than would be expected for your age. It doesn't imply that your ovaries function better than expected for your age or that your chances for conception are any better than the statistics I have previously quoted for your age group. An abnormal result from either of these tests indicates that there is a much lower chance, but not an absolute inability, that you will conceive on your own and deliver a healthy baby.

Abnormal results of FSH testing allow doctors to identify

couples who will be predicted to have a particularly difficult time conceiving. This enables couples to consider medical interventions earlier and, equally importantly, it gives couples with abnormal test results a realistic idea of the difficulties they may have in conceiving.

Each couple is unique, and your doctor may identify specific concerns that need to be addressed before you attempt to conceive on your own. As a couple gets older, their physician will recognize they have a higher potential for general medical or specific fertility problems, and he or she will be more willing to offer testing or treatment sooner.

CONCLUSIONS

Of all the factors affecting fertility, age is one of the most important. Most readers will not or cannot change their plans for starting or expanding their family based on fertility concerns. Within reason, I don't suggest that couples alter their pregnancy plans due to age. It is true, though, that couples over 35, and especially 40 years or older, have special needs and are more likely to have problems.

Although I really believe all women, regardless of age, can get significant benefit from a preconceptional visit to their physician, *I strongly encourage women age 35 and older to see an obstetrician/gynecologist prior to pregnancy for preconceptional counseling.* If a woman is 40 years or older and healthy with normal cycles, I suggest trying for no more than six to nine months before making an appointment with an obstetrician/gynecologist or reproductive endocrinologist for a formal evaluation.

Couples must have realistic expectations regarding their fertility. Optimizing all of the preconceptional recommendations in this book will be extremely valuable for the older couple. No significant interventions can alter the effects of age on your reproductive system; however, the general suggestions made to reduce birth defects, increase fertility, optimize maternal health during pregnancy, and decrease the risk of miscarriage are especially important for the older couple. In addition to following the recommendations outlined in Chapter 3, older couples can obtain screening tests for ovarian function and sperm count to look for any problems in advance of efforts to conceive. Your doctor may also identify other unique concerns based on your own personal history and offer appropriate testing and treatment.

Despite the increased difficulty you may experience, the odds of conceiving naturally and delivering a healthy baby are in your favor at nearly any age until about age forty; however, there is a substantial amount of individual variation. It is appropriate to be optimistic, but your perspective should also be realistic. Taking an organized approach to conception by applying the information in this book will maximize your chances of success.

11
—
Choosing the Sex of Your Baby

If a woman emits semen [then she] . . . bears a man-child.

—*Leviticus 12:2*

THE desire to influence the sex of your baby is a very ancient one. As you can see from the quote above, the Book of Leviticus advocated female orgasm to beget male offspring. The early Greeks, on the other hand, thought that the removal of the left testicle would result in a male child, as they believed boys always came from sperm developed in the right testicle.

Internationally, the overwhelming choice for the sex of a child has traditionally been male. China is a prime example: at one point there were nearly 50 percent more boys born than girls, due to abortions and infanticide.

In contrast, when polled, the majority of American couples prefer girls. There is no single reason for this, but a "family balancing" rationale should lead to a desire for equal numbers of boys and girls. Women often prefer a daughter to share common experiences, as men may favor a son for the same reason. It may be that because women are now able to control their reproduction they are asserting their preferences. One of my patients who already had two boys expresses the feelings of many women: "I love my two boys more than anything in the world, but I hope my next baby is a girl. It's just different. I want us to go shopping together, I can braid her hair, watch her ballet classes . . . things I can't do with my boys."

As I researched information for this chapter I tried to maintain objectivity, but I knew I had my own agenda. My wife, Kara, and I had one child at that point in time, our son, Scott. Kara had said, "I want to keep trying until we have a girl, but if we get to four boys then I'll want to stop." I only have one sibling, an older brother, so I was quite content to have only two kids. This seemed normal to me. Therefore, I was interested in finding a safe, easy, and effective method to increase our odds of having a girl the second time to "balance" our family, to make us both happy, and to stop having kids before I have to trade in our Volvo wagon for a Chevy Suburban.

As it turns out, our second child was also a boy. Because of what you'll read in this chapter, we decided we would not attempt any home methods to influence the sex of our next child. When we conceived again, without any sex-selection intervention, it was a girl.

There are many techniques, both traditional and high-tech, that have been proposed to influence the sex of your child. You can easily spend hours on the Web surfing sites for sex selection techniques, from chat rooms and home pages—with "sure-fire" techniques to try at home—to the Web pages of private fertility clinics offering more technologically sophisticated methods. If you go to your bookstore you will find many authors offering methods to influence the sex of your child. Who should you believe?

After a careful review of the medical literature on sex selection techniques, I will tell you frankly that few, if any, of the popular home methods have any compelling research to support their effectiveness. There are a few sophisticated methods of sex selection with proven benefit. However, the principal purpose of this book is to help you conceive a healthy baby as quickly as possible. Because some of the techniques that can be attempted at home may actually delay your conception, and especially since most of them almost certainly don't work anyway, I would caution against using these techniques if you want to get pregnant on a timetable.

In this chapter I will review the most common methods for sex selection using the latest scientific information and some common sense. Hopefully this will help you decide which techniques, if any, are worth spending your time, effort, and, in some cases, money.

WHAT CAN BE TRIED AT HOME?

My patients and some physicians have many, often creative ideas about techniques that can be used to influence the sex of a baby. These include timing of intercourse, frequency of intercourse, sexual positions, female orgasm, special douching, and nutrition, among others. "My grandmother told me . . ." or "My mother told me . . ." is how the sentences used to begin when patients asked me about techniques to try at home. More recently, the sentences sound more like, "I read on the Internet that [*fill in the blank*] nearly guarantees a boy."

All sex-selection methods depend on the fact that there are two types of sperm: the X-bearing sperm that lead to a female baby, and the Y-bearing sperm that result in a male baby. Most of the recommendations in this section stem from two important hypotheses (I didn't say facts) about these two types of sperm: 1) Male-producing (Y-bearing) sperm swim faster than female sperm, and 2) female-producing (X-bearing) sperm are hardier and last longer than the male sperm.

A number of books have been published on the ways a couple can influence the sex of their child. One of the earlier and better-known books, called *How to Choose the Sex of Your Baby*, was first published in 1970 by Dr. Landrum Shettles and David Rorvik. Their book offers many of the common recommendations such as positions, orgasm, douching, and timing of intercourse. They especially emphasize the timing of intercourse, suggesting that intercourse two to three days before ovulation should favor females, whereas intercourse on the day of ovulation should increase the proportion of males. When a couple combines all of their recommendations, the authors assert, they should have about an 80 percent chance of having a baby of the sex desired.

Let's examine some of the commonly described natural methods that can be tried at home.

Position of Sexual Intercourse

In some cultures the man is traditionally told to make love while lying on his right side in order to assure a son, whereas intercourse on his left side produces a daughter. Traditional ideas such as this one are decried as superstition, but more recent authors make the "scientific" claim that depth of penetration can be used to take advantage of the different swimming speeds of the sperm types. According to this theory, entering from the rear allows deeper penetration, depositing the semen closer to the cervix; this is supposed to favor the faster-swimming male-producing sperm. The other side of the issue, both literally and figuratively, would be that shallow penetration in the "missionary" position would result in deposition of the sperm farther from the cervix and therefore favor the hardier female-producing sperm.

In reality, penile length is usually more than adequate to deposit the sperm up against the cervix regardless of position. Trust me that if it were that easy, someone would have figured it out a long time ago and this chapter would be very short.

Changing Your Vaginal pH

Because some investigators believe the female-producing sperm are more hardy, certain physicians have recommended that women douche before sex to alter their vaginal pH. A high-acidity vaginal environment (low pH) can be accomplished with a vinegar and water douche and is presumed to decrease the numbers of male sperm, since they are supposedly more delicate and more easily damaged by the acid than the female sperm. An alkaline environment (high pH), which would favor the male sperm, can be created by douching with bicarbonate and water.

A study performed by Dr. R. B. Diasio and Dr. Robert Glass, published in the journal *Fertility and Sterility*, found that vaginal pH has no effect on sperm activity. A second study by Dr. P. M. Muehleis and S. Y. Long, also published in *Fertility and Sterility*, confirmed that pH has no effect on sex ratios among the babies born. So it appears that vaginal douching will not influence the sex of your baby. On the other hand, it can be harmful to your vaginal health—as I discussed in Chapter 2— leading to a possible yeast infection or bacterial vaginosis (BV). This condition can definitely increase the rate of preterm labor and probably also increases the rate of miscarriage, pelvic inflammatory disease, and ectopic pregnancy, and delays conception. Due to these possible side effects and the proven lack of effectiveness, I would discourage you from douching prior to sex.

Female Orgasm

If the female partner achieves an orgasm, this is supposed to favor a baby boy. The reason for this theory also relates to vaginal pH, since the female orgasm is supposed to create a more alkaline environment. As stated above, though, pH appears to have no significant effect on sperm activity or resulting sex ratios.

Nutrition

The idea that nutritional alterations could affect sex selection dates back to Chinese yin-yang philosophy. Altering nutrition has been successful in animals, but there is limited information relating to humans. The physiological mechanism involved in animals is not clear. The animal studies would suggest that a diet rich in potassium and sodium, including meats, potatoes, and bananas, while excluding calcium-rich foods such as dairy products, eggs, or greens, results in a higher number of boys; whereas the opposite diet—high in calcium and low in potassium and sodium—increases the ratio in favor of girls. A study by two French researchers, Dr. Joseph Stolkowski and Dr. Jacques Lorrain, published in 1980 evaluated two strict diets of 260 women and the influence of these diets on the sex of their babies. The women began the dietary restrictions during the month prior to attempting to become pregnant, for at least four to six weeks before conception, and continued on the diet until their pregnancy was confirmed.

The diet was very specific about the daily amounts of calcium, magnesium, sodium, and potassium to be consumed. To conceive a girl the mother-to-be had to consume: 1,500 milligrams of calcium, 250 milligrams of magnesium, 675 milligrams of sodium, and 3,000 milligrams of potassium. The women also took an extra 500-milligram calcium tablet with vitamin D each day. To conceive a boy the women consumed a diet high in salt and potassium but low in calcium and magnesium: 300 milligrams of calcium, 135 milligrams of magnesium, 5,000 milligrams of sodium, and 4,000 milligrams of potassium, with an extra tablet of 600 milligrams of potassium chloride once in the morning and once at night.

The doctors claimed a success rate for conceiving a child of the preferred sex greater than 80 percent of the time. Keep in mind that although 260 women sounds like a lot of people, it really isn't in statistical terms. No large-scale studies have been performed in the last twenty years to offer any more insight into this question.

There just is not enough information to be able to say whether there is any merit to dietary alterations or what the specific diet would be. As long as you are taking your prenatal multivitamin and eating a healthy diet, I doubt any harm to you or your baby or any delay in conception would result from trying this method. The investigators did mention certain contraindications to participating in this diet, including hypernervousness, elevated calcium levels, high blood pressure, and kidney problems. Some other problems that would seem to contraindicate this diet are diabetes or a history of cardiovascular disease. I would suggest that if you have any medical problem you contact your doctor to find out if there is any reason to suspect that trying this diet for four to six weeks might be harmful.

If you decide you want to try dietary manipulations, it is much harder than it sounds. You will need to calculate the three meals and snacks for the next day in advance and read all the packages to determine exactly how much of each mineral is in each item. There are also books that can tell you how much of each mineral is normally found in nonpackaged items, such as fruits and vegetables. It might be easier to buy packaged goods, since all of the nutritional information is on the labels.

To facilitate this process I involved a registered dietician, Kelli Hughes, RD, to help readers calculate the mineral contents of common foods. Her tables of food items, and their corresponding levels of potassium, sodium, calcium, and magnesium, are found at the end of the book in Appendix B. If you decide to alter your diet to try and influence the sex of your baby, these tables should help considerably.

Keep in mind that when supplementing your diet with minerals, you are interested in how much "elemental" mineral is in the tablet, not the total milligrams of the tablet. For example, a common brand of calcium citrate comes in 950-milligram tablets, but only 200 milligrams of the tablet is actually elemental calcium. So, if you want to supplement 950 milligrams of calcium, you will need five tablets.

If you find yourself supplementing with extra tablets, make sure you don't go overboard on other nutrients. The potential dangers of megadosing on various nutrients, together with recommended dietary allowances of these nutrients, have been discussed in Chapter 3.

Frequency of Intercourse

According to one theory, frequent intercourse lowers male-sperm counts. Therefore, infrequent intercourse increases the proportion of male offspring. The frequency-method advocates would tell couples to have the man abstain for five days before ovulation (and time intercourse with ovulation) to increase the chances for a boy. Conversely, frequent intercourse—every day—prior to ovulation would increase the chances for a girl.

Some studies have examined abstinence periods and resulting sex ratios. The conclusions of the studies have been mixed, but in all cases the change in percentages of X- and Y-bearing sperm has been minimal in either direction. Regardless of which study is most accurate, the marginal differences do not offer any significant benefit for sex selection. Therefore, attempting to alter the frequency of your intercourse will not help you choose the sex of your baby.

Timing of Intercourse

By far the most common and widely practiced technique for gender determination is timing intercourse in regard to ovulation. Janet, 32, told me her mother had given her very specific instructions: "If you want to have a boy, make him save up and only have sex when you think you're ovulating."

The timing method has been around at least since the 1950s, and proponents, such as Dr. Shettles, believe that intercourse two to three days before ovulation should favor females, whereas intercourse on the day of ovulation should increase the proportion of males. These recommendations are based on the assumption that male-producing sperm are faster swimming but less hardy than the female-producing sperm. So the male-producing sperm get to the egg more quickly, but if the egg is not released during or soon after intercourse, then the female-producing sperm are more likely to survive and fertilize the egg.

Recently I saw a news story on CNN about sex selection. The reporter discussed the commonly held recommendation that having intercourse two to three days in advance of the day of ovulation should favor females, whereas intercourse on the day of ovulation should increase the proportion of males. Next the reporter interviewed a woman with an Internet site for this information and feedback on the success of the method. This woman claimed that 75 percent of her respondents reported success with this method in choosing the sex of their baby.

It occurred to me that this woman's website was a classic example of what statisticians call "reporting bias." In this case, it is likely that the couples who had success with the method were so excited that they wanted to tell everyone how well it worked, so they gave feedback on the website. Those couples who didn't have a baby of the desired sex were obviously less happy with the method and much less likely to spend any time on this site. This is hardly a scientific or reliable way to assess the success of a method.

The formal medical literature does include some recent and high quality research studies designed to examine whether the timing of intercourse affects the sex of a baby. A study in 1995 by Dr. Allen Wilcox, published in the *New England Journal of Medicine*, one of the most highly respected medical sources, examined the relationship between timing of intercourse and the sex of the baby in 136 women. They concluded that no relationship exists between the sex of the baby and timing of intercourse. An earlier article by Dr. Ronald Gray from Johns Hopkins University and colleagues from other institutions, published in *The American Journal of Obstetricians and Gynecologists* in 1991, reviewed six other studies that examined the question of timing of intercourse and sex selection. They concluded that no increase in male offspring occurred with the timing of intercourse at ovulation. In 1989, Dr. P. W. Zarutskie and his colleagues at the University of Washington reviewed all of the pertinent published medical literature on sex selection and timing of intercourse. They published the results in a well-respected, peer-reviewed medical journal called *Fertility and Sterility*. They concluded that there is little if any relationship between the timing of intercourse and sex selection, but if a small association does exist it is actually for a higher percentage of females to be conceived if intercourse occurs close to ovulation. This study, in addition to the others noted above, is in contradiction to the information offered in the well-known book by Dr. Shettles and the similar recommendations by other proponents of a timing method. Dr. Zarutskie's conclusion was that the influence of timing of intercourse on the sex of the resulting baby is quite subtle and is "not a practical method to alter the sex ratio for individual couples." So, it appears that attempts to

Figure 11.1

TIMING OF INTERCOURSE AND SEX SELECTION

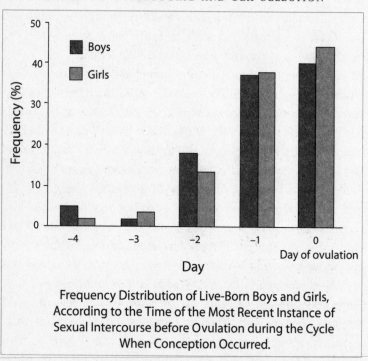

Frequency Distribution of Live-Born Boys and Girls, According to the Time of the Most Recent Instance of Sexual Intercourse before Ovulation during the Cycle When Conception Occurred.

time intercourse with ovulation will not in any significant way increase a couple's chance to determine the sex of their child.

Conclusions Regarding the Methods That Can Be Tried at Home

It appears that home methods for sex selection offer few practical results. The problem is that many couples want a "natural" method to work, so it's difficult to accept that it does not. Additionally, there is a mountain of anecdotal information, mostly in the form of questionnaires, websites, or testimonials, that support many of these techniques—especially regarding timing and frequency of intercourse. As I mentioned earlier, anecdotal information is so fraught with bias that most statisticians would not consider it a reliable form of data.

Some would say that it doesn't hurt couples to think these home methods might work, so let them try. However, this leads to false hopes and wasted money, and it may in some cases delay conception. Once again, common sense tells you that if choosing the sex of your baby were as easy as timing or ejaculatory frequency, many cultures with a strong desire for sex preselection would have put it into practice a long time ago.

Because the main focus of this book is conceiving a healthy baby quickly, I caution you about the use of many of these ineffective home methods. Purposely having intercourse remote from ovulation or using special douches may well prolong the time it takes to conceive. Despite the limited information available, I do not discourage women from trying dietary manipulations because it is possible, although unlikely, that this method is effective.

Although there are no well-accepted methods for sex selection that can be used at home, there are more sophisticated methods offered at some fertility specialists' offices and a few select medical centers. Some of these techniques have been proven to be unreliable, others are controversial, but a few of the methods are now accepted as effective.

SOPHISTICATED (HIGH-TECH) SEX-SELECTION TECHNIQUES

The most basic laboratory technique, and one of the oldest, consists of allowing the sperm to swim through various media (fluids) designed to separate the male-producing sperm from the female-producing sperm. Probably the best recognized of these techniques is called the Ericsson method, or Gametrics. In 1973, Dr. Ronald Ericsson reported a method by which he could concentrate the "male" sperm up to 85 percent, or to a lesser extent concentrate the "female" sperm, by making the sperm swim through albumin (a type of protein). Nowadays, proponents of Dr. Ericsson's method claim effectiveness greater than or equal to 75 percent, and the cost ranges between $600 and $1,100. These fees are not covered by any insurance companies.

About 30 U.S. and numerous international clinics offer the Ericsson method. Despite this fact, the technique has failed to be validated, and the American College of Obstetricians and Gynecologists (ACOG), the largest organization representing obstetrician/gynecologists in the United States, formed a "Committee Opinion" in November 1996 regarding sex-selection techniques. This document stated, "No current techniques for prefertilization sex selection have been shown to be reliable."

Dr. Alan DeCherney, chairman of the department of obstetrics and gynecology at the University of California, Los Angeles, and editor of the medical journal *Fertility and Sterility*, agreed with the ACOG opinion regarding techniques such as the Ericsson method and recommendations for methods of sex selection that can be tried at home when he was quoted in *The New York Times Magazine* as saying, "They don't work, nothing works." You should certainly keep these quotes in mind if you ever consider buying a book on home methods of sex selection or paying a physician a fee to use one of these sperm separation methods.

PROVEN SOPHISTICATED (HIGH-TECH) METHODS FOR SEX SELECTION

There are definitely some techniques that are well accepted as significantly increasing your chances for selecting the sex of your child. The bad news is that the techniques are expensive and high-technology, require a visit to a very limited number of centers around the world, and may involve an uncertain amount of risk.

Flow Cytometry/MicroSort

The newest and most promising method is called flow cytometry, and is quite a bit more sophisticated and complicated than the Ericsson-type techniques. Flow cytometry was first developed by the U.S. Department of Agriculture (USDA) for sorting sperm in farm animals. The flow cytometry machine works by separating female-producing sperm, which weigh slightly more (the X chromosome is bigger than the Y chromosome), from male-producing sperm.

In this method, the flow cytometry machine first dyes the sperm and then strikes the dyed sperm with a laser as the sperm passes through a small opening. The larger "female" sperm give off a higher signal from the laser strike. The two different signals are measured by a machine, which then separates the sperm according to difference in signals. The method works well according to the initial data from farm animals, and the offspring conceived by this technique appear normal.

In the early 1990s, a fertility clinic in Fairfax, Virginia, the Genetics and IVF Institute, obtained a license from the USDA to try to use the flow cytometry machine for sorting sperm in humans. They trademarked the technique as MicroSort. Human male-producing and female-producing sperm only differ in size by about 3 percent, significantly less than the sperm differences in most farm animals, making flow cytometry more difficult to perform in humans.

A clinical trial was launched at the Genetics and IVF Institute in 1993, and by 1995 the first MicroSort baby was born. To be included in the study, couples needed to demonstrate a family or personal history of an X-linked genetic disorder. (X-linked disorders affect only the male offspring, so preselecting female babies allows these couples to have children free of the disease.) This was a medical justification for using the technology, avoiding many of the obvious ethical issues that would present themselves for other couples. Since that time, the eligibility for undergoing the MicroSort technique has expanded to include family balancing, but the couple must already have another child, and the sex selected must be different from the sex of the previous child or children. The cost of the MicroSort treatment is approximately $3,500 per attempt. On average it takes three attempts to become pregnant but that depends on the woman's age and the overall fertility of the couple.

I spoke to a representative of the Genetics and IVF Institute to have the most recent update of their statistics at the end of

2005. They reported that the technique was about 90 percent successful for choosing females. The MicroSort technique does not do as well at selecting males. It is approximately 76 percent successful at choosing male babies. So far, of the approximately 700 babies delivered after MicroSort treatment there were no apparent adverse effects from the sperm-separation technique. Although promising, it is too early to say whether this method will prove to be reliable and safe in large groups of children and after extended follow-up.

Preimplantation Genetic Diagnosis

There is one sex selection technique, called Preimplantation Genetic Diagnosis (PGD), that is virtually 100 percent accurate; but it is very expensive, highly technical, and requires that you undergo a treatment of in vitro fertilization (IVF). In general, the couples offered this testing for sex determination are only those with a personal or family history of a serious congenital sex-linked disease, in which the gene for the disease appears on the Y chromosome. For those couples who require IVF for other reasons (for instance, tubal blockage or low sperm count), PGD is not routinely performed because it has not been proven to improve pregnancy rates, adds expense, and, perhaps, risks damaging the embryos in the process. PGD may be offered to couples undergoing IVF who have recurrent miscarriages, a personal or family history of some genetic diseases, advanced maternal age, or recurrent failure of IVF treatments. In these cases, some IVF clinics will provide information regarding the sex of the embryos. However, most IVF programs have decided against allowing couples to choose the sex of the embryos that will be placed in the uterus due to the ethical concerns involved.

Ultrasound and Sex Selection

We have reviewed selection methods to be used before fertilization or implantation of the early baby into the uterus. I should also mention another technique that involves the use of ultrasound for pregnant women at the end of the first trimester. By about 12 weeks of gestation, an ultrasound can usually determine the sex of a fetus.

A few physicians in the United States are willing to perform an ultrasound for pregnant women at about 12 weeks of gestation, for a fee, with the assumption that couples who do not have a fetus of the desired sex will undergo an elective abortion. The most infamous practitioner is Dr. John Stephens, self-described as "the most hated physician in America." This practice is universally considered unethical by the American medical community. However, it is much more common and accepted outside the United States, in countries such as India or China.

Ethical Issues

I don't think this section would be complete if I did not at least briefly mention the ethical issues involved in sex preselection. Unless the couple is trying to avoid sex-chromosome-linked genetic disease, ethicists agree that sex selection is purely a selfish desire by the parents, because choosing the gender offers no benefits to a child. Sex selection inherently reflects the idea that the sex of a child makes that child more or less valued. In many cultures in the world, systematic sex preferences come from the underlying inequalities between the sexes. Ethicists worry that sex selection perpetuates these inequalities. It's not hard to imagine some of the possible problems that could be created globally if someone came up with a simple, cheap, effective technique for sex selection.

The question of whether it is ethically or morally right for members of a society to choose the sex of their baby is not something I want to try to answer here in this book. You may be thinking, "My one child wouldn't make much of a difference—after all, there are six billion people on this planet." However, this question is not just a personal one, because on a larger scale it has profound implications for our society and the global population. I'll leave this complex issue for you to ponder while the search continues for a practical method. There is no doubt that in the near future there will be cheap, effective, and easily accessible methods for sex selection. Then these ethical issues will no longer be merely theoretical.

CONCLUSIONS

There are only a few ways to reliably choose the sex of your baby: preimplantation genetic diagnosis, late first trimester ultrasound with a possible abortion, and flow cytometry. Preimplantation diagnosis is not going to be an option for the vast majority of readers. I sincerely hope that none of my readers would consider finding a practitioner to provide an ultrasound followed by an abortion if the baby is not of the desired sex. So, it appears that for family balancing, the only method that might be worth investing your time, money, or effort in is flow cytometry, and the only licensed method at the present time is called MicroSort, currently offered at a few clinics in the United States. Additionally, the technique appears to be more successful in selecting girls.

The effectiveness of dietary therapy is unlikely to be high, but its success rate is uncertain due to a lack of studies. If you want to try it, make sure to take your daily prenatal vitamin to protect against birth defects. Appendix B will help you to get organized with the dietary restrictions. With respect to other home methods of sex selection and the other techniques offered at some fertility clinics, most evidence indicates that they offer little practical benefit in choosing the sex of your child.

Before researching the subject I thought that my obstetrics and gynecology residency had exposed me to enough babies with birth defects to convince me that the health of the baby was all that mattered. And perhaps equally powerful was the experience I had in my infertility fellowship, working with couples who had spent years of their lives and huge emotional and financial investments just trying to become pregnant. I surprised myself while writing this chapter, when I did allow myself to consider the possibility of using a sex selection technique to help assure that our next baby is a girl.

After my wife, Kara, read my rough draft of this chapter, we talked specifically about MicroSort. It would be an easy trip up from our home (at that time) in North Carolina. Kara is actually from Fairfax, Virginia, the home of the Genetics and IVF Institute, and I'm from the next town over, so we could attend the clinic and visit some of our friends and family in the area. Because we want a girl, the method would provide us an excellent chance of success.

We decided that sex selection isn't something we want. Central to Kara's decision was her concern about the uncertain level of risk involved. She told me, "If there was a reliable, natural way, and we weren't fooling with nature with all this technology, I might actually try it." We decided that if we did the MicroSort technique and twenty years from now researchers found that the flow cytometry method led to an increased risk for cancer or some other serious disease, we wouldn't be able to live with ourselves if our child became affected. We also decided that in this Information Age we are all trying to better understand and control our world, but maybe there are a few things we should still leave to chance.

Obviously many couples feel differently than Kara and I do, as evidenced by the popularity of MicroSort. Studies have shown that as many as one-quarter of the U.S. population would try a sex selection method if it were safe, effective, and inexpensive. I foresee that a method that fulfills all of the necessary requirements will become widely available in the relatively near future. As Dr. Benjamin Younger, executive director of the American Society of Reproductive Medicine, said, "People want it. And when people want things, science finds a way to make it happen."

Sex selection, coming soon to a clinic near you . . . .

12

—

When Nature Needs a Boost:
What to Expect from a Fertility Doctor

WHEN TO GO?

I recommend that all couples see their family practitioner or obstetrician/gynecologist for a preconceptional counseling visit. In a perfect world, all couples would have the recommended testing, counseling, and interventions noted in Chapter 3, "Preconceptional Care." Well-informed readers can help their clinician concentrate on the important issues addressed in Chapter 3, some of which may be unique to each couple.

This chapter focuses on what couples should expect from a visit with a doctor or other professional beyond preconceptional counseling if they are having problems becoming pregnant or if they have some concerns about how difficult it may be to become pregnant. But when should you go see a professional?

As a general rule, infertility is defined as the inability to conceive after one year of unprotected, regular intercourse. As far as I can tell, this is an arbitrarily chosen time frame. Without a doubt, if you have been trying for a year without success, you should make an appointment with your physician or other caregiver. But you do not have to wait a year. Let us apply some common sense to this question of when to seek professional help. For instance, if you have irregular menstrual cycles, or another issue that would be expected to interfere with your ability to conceive in a reasonable time frame, then you should have met with your practitioner for a preconceptional visit even before trying to conceive.

I never cease to be amazed by the patients who tell me their practitioner wanted them to try for an entire year before any testing or treatment would be offered. This is despite circumstances such as the woman having no menstrual periods at all (amenorrhea), polycystic ovarian syndrome, or a previous history of infertility requiring treatment to become pregnant! Although unintentional, comments by practitioners such as, "You'll never know if you'll have a problem until you try," are often interpreted by patients as dismissive. Sometimes you have to be your own advocate. If the recommendation doesn't make sense, then let your practitioner know that you would like to start an evaluation and ask for a referral, or refer yourself. Many insurance companies do not require a referral to a reproductive endocrinologist. Others will require it, so you need to contact your insurance company to find out.

Figure 12.1

COMMON REASONS FOR EARLY REFERRAL TO A FERTILITY SPECIALIST (LESS THAN 1 YEAR OF TRYING TO CONCEIVE)

- Age 35 or older
- History of difficulty becoming pregnant with previous conception(s)
- History of more than one pregnancy loss
- Irregular menstrual cycles
- History of polycystic ovarian syndrome (PCOS) (see Chapter 2)

- History of endometriosis (see Chapter 2)
- Partner with history of infertility with a previous partner
- Either partner with medical problems (or history) that might affect fertility (for example: either partner with history of radiation or chemotherapy, female with history of pelvic surgery or pelvic infection)
- Family history of early menopause

WHO TO SEE?

Some family practitioners, nurse practitioners, internists, and other caregivers are comfortable with starting an evaluation. However, most are not and will refer you to an obstetrician/ gynecologist (ob/gyn) or a fertility specialist, referred to as a reproductive endocrinologist. Some ob/gyns are more interested in infertility or have received more training than others. Therefore, ob/gyns provide varying levels of infertility testing and treatment. When to consult a fertility specialist (reproductive endocrinologist) depends on both your and your practitioner's level of confidence and comfort. Depending on the underlying problem, it is very common and quite acceptable for couples to start the evaluation and treatment with their family practitioner or obstetrician/gynecologist.

What's the difference between an ob/gyn and a reproductive endocrinologist? An ob/gyn is a physician who completes a four-year residency program in obstetrics and gynecology. Like the ob/gyn, the reproductive endocrinologist also completed a four-year residency program in obstetrics and gynecology. However, the reproductive endocrinologist was selected to complete an additional three-year fellowship in reproductive endocrinology and infertility. This fellowship involves the medical and surgical aspects of all types of problems affecting infertile couples. This is the only group of specialists subspecialty trained and certified to work with infertile couples. Other practitioners who advertise as "fertility specialists" or offer "infertility care" are obviously interested in this issue and may have practical experience, but they have no additional training or special certification to provide this care.

Also, don't confuse a "medical endocrinologist" with a "reproductive endocrinologist"; they are different. A medical endocrinologist is an internist who specializes in problems such as thyroid disease and diabetes and does not receive the specialized training required for certification to care for infertile couples.

Another important factor to consider is that all couples have a limited amount of emotional reserve. If the time to become pregnant is long enough, every couple will eventually reach a point where they are out of energy and cannot weather the disappointment any longer. Some will run out of energy before they ever reach the fertility specialist. Unfortunately, they discontinue therapy before they receive the most effective treatment. Practically speaking, financial reserve is another problem. Unless you have good infertility insurance, you may find that you have exhausted your savings before reaching your goal of becoming pregnant. I am obviously biased, but if you have a reproductive endocrinologist in your area, I suggest you go straight to him or her.

Who are the reproductive endocrinologists in your area? Your ob/gyn will always know, because they refer patients all the time. There may also be multiple practices in your area, and your ob/gyn can give you some advice as to which one they recommend. The yellow pages should list specialists in your area. Look under physicians—sometimes they are found in the infertility section, other times in the ob/gyn section. The American Society for Reproductive Medicine also has a website to help identify providers in your area at *www.asrm.org*, as does the Society for Reproductive Endocrinology and Infertility (SREI) at *www.SREI.org*.

Another good source of information is Resolve (The National Infertility Association), an influential infertility advocacy group in the United States. Resolve recommends that when a couple requires more than basic treatment with clomiphene citrate to stimulate ovulation, it is in your best interest to establish care with a specialist in reproductive endocrinology and infertility. I encourage you to visit their website at *www.resolve.org* for more information and links to other useful websites.

To be thorough, even reproductive endocrinologists have levels to their certification. After completing their fellowship training, most reproductive endocrinologists take both a written and an oral examination given on separate years. Once they have passed the written exam, physicians must then complete an oral examination given only once a year in Dallas, Texas. If they pass both these exams, they become subspecialty certified in reproductive endocrinology and infertility. Only two-thirds to three-quarters of the physicians who take the oral exam each year pass and obtain this certification.

Physicians who complete their fellowship are not required to take these exams or pass them, and physicians can practice all aspects of reproductive endocrinology and infertility without being certified. So you should not assume your physician is certified. It is perfectly reasonable to find out if your physician is "subspecialty certified" before making an appointment. Usually it will be posted on their website. You can also call their office to ask, or find out if they are a member of the Society for Reproductive Endocrinology and Infertility (SREI). Only subspecialty-certified reproductive endocrinologists can be full members. Visit the SREI at *www.SREI.org* to find lists of members in your area. You can also learn about a doctor's credentials by contacting the American Board of Medical Specialties (847) 491-9091 or visiting the websites *www.ama-assn.org* or *www.medseek.com*.

Figure 12.2
QUESTIONS TO ASK A FERTILITY SPECIALIST'S OFFICE
BEFORE SCHEDULING AN INITIAL APPOINTMENT

- Is the practice open seven days a week for necessary treatments and procedures?
- Is your insurance accepted by the office? What will your insurance cover? Are there payment plans or other financial details you should be aware of?
- Is the physician subspecialty trained and certified in reproductive endocrinology and infertility?
- Does the practice offer all levels of service, including in vitro fertilization (IVF)?
- How many physicians are in the practice? Will you be able to establish an ongoing relationship with one doctor, or will several share your case?
- Does the physician offer advanced surgical techniques to evaluate and treat infertility?
- If necessary, where would surgery be performed, and at which hospital?

HOW CAN I PREPARE?

This book should give you a good foundation when you meet with a physician or other caregiver for the first time. By definition, "it takes two to tango" when making a baby, so the couple should always go to the appointment together. Fortunately, most couples understand that nearly half the time it is a male problem, or a combined problem for both the male and female. It many cases it makes little sense for me to talk to just one partner when we are doing the initial evaluation.

It is always a good idea to make sure any of your pertinent records are at the doctor's office before your visit. Request all of the office records. If you have had a hysterosalpingogram (X-ray dye study of the pelvis), have a copy of the films forwarded. You should request copies if any other radiological procedure (such as MRI, CT, pelvic ultrasound) was performed and interpreted as abnormal. If you have had a pelvic surgery in the past, you will want to make sure a copy of the operative report is sent. This may be obtained either by requesting a copy from the surgeon's office or from the hospital where it was performed.

Call the office well in advance of your appointment to make sure they have received the records. Some hospitals or doctors' offices take two weeks or more to forward records and will not be rushed, regardless of when you have an appointment. Do not assume when someone says "I'll mail them" or "I'll fax them" that it was done. I strongly suggest that you also request a second copy of your records be sent to your home address. It allows you to have confirmation that everything has been sent, gives you the opportunity to look through your records, and enables you to bring them with you to the first appointment, in case the records never made it to the doctor's office, for whatever reason. Remember, these are your records and you have a right to see them at your written request.

Preparing a brief (one page or less) summary is also useful. It helps to assure your doctor has a clear understanding about your history and refreshes your memory. Patients often tell me they are surprised to see what is in their medical records. Although every caregiver intends to fully inform their patients, practitioners may forget to relay some information, or perhaps the explanation given to the patient is not entirely clear.

Many couples are referred to me after having testing and treatment at their referring doctor's office. They are relieved to be at a specialist's office and have high expectations that during the first visit we will discuss the underlying problem and weigh the options to correct it. Without the records to review, I often have to tell couples that I really need to look at the records first before I can offer my recommendations. This can be frustrating for the couple and for me. Requesting and reviewing records and then exchanging phone messages wastes time. Sometimes it requires an additional office visit to discuss the medical record review. So, if any testing or treatment has been done prior to a referral, you will facilitate the process by making sure all pertinent information is available.

WHAT WILL HAPPEN?

At the first visit to an ob/gyn or reproductive endocrinologist the physician will want to take a detailed history from both partners. Any records will be reviewed. A physical exam will be completed. Often a screening vaginal probe ultrasound is performed immediately following the physical exam. Once the examination is over, the physician will usually sit down with the couple and discuss a plan.

Depending on the couple's history and the findings on the physical exam, a few screening tests are usually suggested. In more than half of the cases, the cause of infertility can be explained by one of three tests: a hysterosalpingogram, a semen analysis, and an evaluation of ovulation. The way I usually explain it to couples is that there are three main issues. Are there enough functional sperm? Is the egg working well and is it being released regularly? Can the sperm and egg find each other?

Sperm

The semen analysis is usually the first suggested test. It is relatively cheap, there are no side effects—apart from a little bit of embarrassment perhaps—and it is revealing in up to 40 percent of cases. Interestingly, it is difficult, if not impossible, to predict the results of a semen analysis. A man's "young and healthy" condition has no relationship to his semen analysis. Dr. R. S. Lucidi and colleagues published a study, in the journal *Fertility and Sterility* in 2005, which showed that a history of previously fathering a child did not predict that a man's semen analysis result would be normal. Sperm production by the testicles can change. A man can have a perfectly normal semen analysis one year, and the next year the semen analysis can be severely abnormal. Nearly all men need a semen analysis at the initial visit.

What can lead to an abnormal semen analysis result? Many men have a genetic predisposition to poor sperm production. This cannot be improved in most cases. Other men can initially have normal sperm production but can develop a problem. Men can develop swollen veins around the testicle(s), called a varicocele, which is usually unnoticeable by the man. This is a similar phenomenon to varicose veins in the legs but occurs in the scrotum. The dilated, enlarged veins increase the testicular temperature, which may significantly reduce sperm production. Inflammation and infection in the male genital tract can dramatically affect sperm production. Illnesses, such as some common viruses, can also temporarily lower sperm production. In some cases, exposure to environmental toxins, known or unknown, can be a problem. The disappearance of the exposure may also explain the return of normal semen parameters. The best example of this is smoking cessation. Poor nutrition has also been associated with abnormal semen parameters. Remember that sperm take approximately 72 days to be produced, so it may take two to three months before sperm production will normalize once a problem has been corrected.

Referral to a urologist is usually suggested if a semen analysis is found to be significantly abnormal. I always suggest that a second semen analysis be performed prior to the referral to the urologist. It is not uncommon to find that, although the first semen analysis had some problems, the second semen analysis returns normal. I usually explain to couples, "he probably had a bad day" the first time. If this is the case I do suggest a third semen analysis to further evaluate.

This "bad day" phenomenon is real and was illustrated nicely by a study by Dr. C. A. Paulsen of one "normal" man who gave sperm samples every other week for two years and four months. Considering a normal sperm count is 20 million per milliliter of semen or greater, the man had quite variable concentrations. He gave a total of 115 samples, and his sperm counts ranged from 1 million per milliliter, to 170 million per milliliter during the greater than two-year period. Usually the results were normal at 20 million per milliliter or greater (115 times), but on five occasions he had abnormal counts ranging from only 1 million per milliliter to 12 million per milliliter. If you happened to have caught him on one of these "bad days" he would be suspected of having a fertility problem. The takeaway message is: don't panic over a single abnormal semen analysis result. If it is abnormal, do a second one.

Some fertility specialists have all men do two semen analyses. This is a good strategy. However, to be cost-effective and minimize the number of trips to my office, if the first analysis looks perfectly normal, I don't usually ask men to repeat another analysis within a year. It seems unlikely that a man who usually has quite poor semen parameters would coincidentally be able to provide a perfectly normal sample the day of his semen analysis. Although unlikely, this is possible, so if you want to rule this out completely, proceed with two semen analyses.

Interpreting a semen analysis can actually be somewhat complicated. It isn't as simple as we have assumed. The long-standing criteria for a semen analysis were created by the World Health Organization (WHO) many years ago. The WHO defines a normal semen analysis when it meets the following criteria:

Semen volume > 1.5 mL
Sperm concentration > 20 million/mL
Motility (swimming ability) > 50 percent
Morphology (shape of sperm) > 50 percent normal

In 2001, Dr. Guzick and colleagues published probably the best study evaluating what the result of a semen analysis indicates in terms of predicting the fertility of a man, in the *New England Journal of Medicine*. Unfortunately, the results of the study revealed that it is not as simple as has been assumed by the WHO system. The modern interpretation of a semen analysis now recognizes an "indeterminate zone" for numbers of motile sperm. Sperm concentrations between 13.5 million per milliliter and 48 million per milliliter and motility between 32 percent and 63 percent are broad "indeterminate" areas. Men in these ranges may be more or less fertile. If the levels are below these (13.5 million/mL and 32 percent motile), it is clearly predictive of infertility. Levels higher than these ranges (48 million/mL and 63 percent motile) are considered normal.

The more modern semen analysis that has been widely adopted by fertility specialists and their laboratories also involves a different morphology assessment than the WHO criteria. It is called the Kruger "strict" morphology, named after

Dr. Thinus Kruger from South Africa. This system describes only the percentage of perfectly shaped sperm. This morphology system is better at predicting fertility than the old WHO criteria. Normal is greater than or equal to 12 percent, subfertile is less than 9 percent. When the morphology is less than 4 percent this appears to be particularly concerning. That leaves an "indeterminate zone" of 4 to 11 percent. Many men fall between 4 and 11 percent, and some of these men will show normal fertility but others will be infertile. This wide "indeterminate zone" is the major drawback of this system. But when a man has a "strict" morphology of 3 percent or less, it is clearly indicative of problems. Keep in mind that even when the morphology is 0 percent, it never means that a man cannot father a child, but it does indicate that the chances per cycle are quite low.

Now that I've worn you out with the details of a semen analysis, I'm going to tell you that, unfortunately, the results of a standard semen analysis do not evaluate the sperm as completely as once thought. We have been letting men "off the hook" for decades, telling them their "sperm count is normal." It turns out that this is a vast oversimplification. In reality, some men with perfectly normal semen analyses are infertile. How can that be possible?

Sperm are basically a package of DNA with a tail to push that DNA through the female genital tract, up to an egg, through the egg's "shell," and finally into the cytoplasm to cause fertilization. Sometimes the sperm numbers (count), the swimming ability (motility), and the appearance (morphology) are all normal, but the DNA inside is significantly damaged. If the DNA is significantly damaged, the sperm may have difficulty providing the genetic information necessary to allow formation of a normal embryo.

There are a number of tests commercially available now to assess DNA damage. The most common one is the sperm chromatin structure assay (SCSA). Should you ask your doctor for a sperm DNA test initially? At this point in time, my answer is no in most circumstances. Unfortunately, the tests for DNA damage are not perfected yet. The level of DNA damage may predict lower fertility, but there does not appear to be an absolute cutoff where a physician can say that the sperm are not capable of fertilizing an egg. For this reason, most fertility programs do not offer this test initially. In many circumstances it tends to create more anxiety than insight. In my experience, for couples who are getting started with an infertility evaluation and treatment plan, the results of a DNA damage assessment rarely, if ever, change my initial recommendations.

It's important also to keep in mind my recommendations from Chapter 8, "The Man's Role in Getting Pregnant Quickly." I encourage all men to take the vitamin supplements and make the lifestyle changes that would be expected to improve sperm DNA quality. These suggestions are exactly the ones I give to men who have high levels of DNA damage discovered when tested. So instead of testing everyone and only treating those with high levels of DNA damage, I recommend empirically treating all men, whether they have the testing or not.

We have been misled for decades that a "normal" semen analysis (by WHO criteria) meant that the male partner was fine and the female partner must be the one with the problem. Unfortunately, there are still many practitioners who have this mind-set. In fact, most doctors who are not reproductive endocrinologists are not aware of the implications of abnormal sperm morphology or sperm DNA testing. I am quite certain that new tests of sperm function and DNA damage will be available in the future that are better than the existing ones. Undoubtedly, we will learn that other subgroups of men have DNA damage, or other problems leading to sperm dysfunction, that we cannot detect with the present tests available. For this reason, I take the perspective that all men can improve sperm quality, regardless of whether or not the semen analysis is "normal." Stopping bad habits and taking supplemental vitamins and minerals will likely produce higher quality sperm. All men should follow these recommendations, regardless of the result of the semen analysis.

Egg

For the woman, one of the first things the practitioner will want to establish is whether or not you are ovulating regularly. This can usually be established merely by talking about the pattern of menstrual bleeding. At your first visit, it is quite helpful to have available a menstrual calendar, basal body temperature charts, or simply a summary of the lengths of at least the last few menstrual cycles. Many couples are using urinary ovulation-prediction kits, urinary monitors, or other modalities to determine the day of ovulation. This is also important information to help define the length of the luteal phase.

Even if your cycles are "like a clock," the doctor will probably want to confirm your ovulation. The most common test to assess ovulation is a serum progesterone measurement. Progesterone only rises measurably following ovulation, so it is an excellent way to objectively evaluate ovulation. The most common way to do this is to have you return in the mid-luteal phase for a serum progesterone measurement.

Progesterone peaks about 7 days after ovulation. Sometimes you will be asked to come between cycle days 21 to 24 for this test. As you learned in Chapter 5, "Timing Is Everything: Predicting Ovulation," this is an oversimplification. However, if your cycle is fairly close to 28 days apart, that is close enough. If your cycle is not close to 28 days apart, mention this to your practitioner. They will appreciate you reminding them, and they should alter the day to return accordingly.

Egg quality is another, much more subtle, issue. I introduced this concept in Chapter 10, "Turning Back the Clock: Getting Pregnant at 35 and Older." Apart from making sure the egg is being released every month, the quality of the egg is obviously very important. This is a much more difficult parameter to ascertain. Egg quality is most commonly affected by age. Although new sperm are being made every day, no more eggs are produced after a woman's birth. Eggs suffer from the effects of aging like all other cell types in the body, such as skin, heart, and skeletal muscles.

Formal testing for egg quality, also referred to as "ovarian reserve" testing, is limited at the present time. This is particularly true for women who making their first fertility-related visit to their practitioner's office and have not had the other basic tests performed (hysterosalpingogram, semen analysis, ultrasound, physical exam, progesterone measurement) or women who have not been trying for more than one year. The most common screening tests of "ovarian reserve" include an antral follicle count and a well-timed blood measurement of follicle stimulating hormone and estradiol. A clomiphene citrate challenge test (CCCT) is a more complicated test to assess ovarian reserve. Other tests exist, such as blood measurements of inhibin B and mullerian inhibiting factor levels, or gonadotropin releasing hormone stimulation testing. These other tests are not very useful yet to predict outcomes and should be considered research tools at the present time.

For couples meeting with me for the first time, I combine a vaginal probe ultrasound with the physical exam. The ultrasound allows me to obtain an antral follicle count. Premenopausally, all women have some "resting" or "antral" follicles in the ovaries. These represent small, normal cysts, called follicles, that each contain an egg. The number of antral follicles gives a fairly good understanding of the function of the ovaries and, indirectly, the quality of the eggs. In general, a low antral follicle count encourages me to consider blood testing for ovarian reserve screening. A normal antral follicle count reassures me that poor ovarian reserve (egg quality) is probably not the central issue. Whether or not to order other egg quality/ovarian reserve testing at your first visit is a discussion to have with your practitioner. Each case should be individualized. Older age tends to be the most important factor motivating me to recommend these tests. In general, though, if the antral follicle count by ultrasound is normal, or if the woman is less than 35 years old, I often discourage it initially for couples. The reason is that the majority of the tests described above were researched and developed for women who have unexplained infertility (other fertility problems have been excluded), and often the couples enrolled in studies failed medical therapies. In many of the research studies the patients were limited to those treated with in vitro fertilization (IVF), and the results of FSH testing or the CCCT were used to predict the success of IVF. Also, research shows the predictive value of FSH testing is lower in younger women.

There is limited research regarding whether to offer FSH testing to women who are "subfertile" and who are just meeting their fertility specialist for the first time. One of the best studies was from Dr. Joris van Montfrans and colleagues, published in the journal *Fertility and Sterility* in 2000. They performed FSH testing on women who were new patients in their clinic desiring to become pregnant, and all had regular menstrual cycles. The women with abnormal FSH testing were compared to age-matched women (controls) who had normal FSH levels. There was no difference in pregnancy rates, time to pregnancy, or miscarriage rates. The conclusion was that "screening for elevated basal FSH concentrations is of no additional value in a general subfertility population with ovulatory menstrual cycles."

Therefore, it is difficult to apply the FSH testing to all women who are visiting a fertility specialist for the first time. Selecting the correct women to have the test is quite important. At the first visit, some women do have a history or findings on examination that suggest FSH testing will be helpful. But I don't order it routinely. If ordered at the wrong time, or for the wrong patient, it isn't a test that is predictive of success or failure, and can create undue anxiety. I suggest you talk to your doctor about how they will interpret and apply the result of the test before it is ordered.

CAN THE SPERM AND EGG GET TOGETHER?

It is important to learn about the internal anatomy of the Fallopian tubes and uterus and discover whether the tubes are open. Unfortunately, the pelvic examination and the ultrasound are quite poor at identifying women with blockage in a Fallopian tube or an abnormal intrauterine cavity. The best way to get information about both the Fallopian tubes and the uterine cavity is by an X-ray dye study called a hysterosalpingogram, or HSG. It is an old-fashioned test, but no other imaging study has ever been able to replace it. The HSG is a very common radiologic procedure performed after menstrual bleeding has ended but before ovulation is expected. During this test contrast material (radio-opaque dye) is introduced into the uterus and Fallopian tubes while a series of X-ray films are taken. It shows the outline of the uterine cavity and the internal anatomy of the Fallopian tubes. If the tubes are open at the end, the dye will spill out and into the pelvis. It is a safe procedure. There is a much less than a 1 percent risk of infection following the procedure, and the rare infection appears to be more common in women who have a blocked and dilated Fallopian tube or tubes. I treat women who have blockage and dilatation of at least one tube at the time of HSG with an antibiotic for one week following the procedure. Otherwise there does not seem to be any compelling research to suggest that antibiotic treatment is necessary for women who have the HSG performed.

The HSG has a reputation for causing discomfort or pain. In my experience it is mostly, but not completely, a holdover from a time in the past when HSGs were performed with a metal apparatus that was quite uncomfortable. Many, but not all, practices have stopped using the old apparatus and now use a flexible plastic balloon catheter that is much more comfortable. You might want to ask your doctor how they are going to do it. Some practitioners, still using the old method, will write patients a prescription for a narcotic pain medication to take prior to the HSG. If this is the case, then you will need someone to drive you home, and you probably need to take at least part of the day off.

Many of my patients will go on-line the night before the procedure to learn about it. Despite my reassurance about the more modern technique, they read horror stories of how bad the procedure is, and they come in fearful about what they will experience. Fortunately, most are underwhelmed by the procedure and say, "It was much better than I thought," or "That wasn't bad." There is a small group who do have significant cramping with the more modern procedure, and despite the gentler technique they have a bad experience. Because you won't know if you'll be in this minority group with significant cramping, I suggest all women take 600 to 800 milligrams of ibuprofen (with a snack or meal) an hour or two before the procedure. You should not require the day off and will be able to return to work afterward.

What Are Some Other Tests That May Be Ordered?

There are a few other tests that used to be commonly ordered but have fallen out of favor in the recent past. Each has been shown to offer limited, if any, useful clinical information. I mention these tests because many couples ask about them, expecting they will be ordered. These include the postcoital test, the endometrial biopsy (when used to diagnose luteal phase problems), and antisperm antibodies in the female partner.

For more than 50 years, a timed endometrial biopsy was commonly undertaken to assess the lining of uterus. It was most often performed to rule out luteal phase deficiency. Dr. Christos Coutifaris and colleagues published a landmark study in 2004 in the journal *Fertility and Sterility*. It was a well-designed, multi-center, NIH-supported study that reported that the endometrial biopsy offered no clinically useful information regarding a woman's fertility. This was a shock to fertility specialists, who had always assumed this test was reliable. The endometrial biopsy went from a very commonly utilized infertility test to a rare test (for this indication) almost overnight.

A postcoital test used to be a commonly performed test, ostensibly to evaluate the sperm-cervical mucus interaction. This was an unusual test wherein the doctor asks the couple to have intercourse before the female partner comes in to be examined. A speculum is inserted and a swab of the cervical mucus was put on a slide to be examined under the microscope. Sperm numbers, swimming ability in the mucus, and the appearance of the mucus could be assessed.

When the results of the postcoital test were abnormal, terms like "hostile cervical mucus" were mentioned, giving the impression of a serious struggle occurring on a microscopic level. It turns out that whether the result of a postcoital test was normal or abnormal, it had limited, if any, predictive value for whether or not you can become pregnant. It also has been shown to be a poor way to assess sperm and cannot replace a formal semen analysis. Therefore, most practitioners have abandoned the postcoital test.

Antisperm antibodies are also an issue that generates questions from my patients. The idea is that antibodies can be a problem when they bind to the sperm. This can lead to reduced motility and damage to the sperm and may cause infertility. Antisperm antibodies come in two types. A man makes antibodies against his own sperm, or the female partner can make antibodies against a male partner's sperm.

Most labs associated with a fertility specialist will offer antisperm antibody testing as part of the semen analysis. So, this is a test that looks at antibodies in the semen that the male has made against his own sperm. The sperm are normally protected from the body's immune system by what is referred to as the "blood-testes-barrier." This barrier can be breached by trauma, surgery, or infection, exposing the immune system to sperm and leading to antibody formation. This can be a useful test and can be predictive of problems, depending on the type of antibodies found and where they are bound to the sperm.

Testing for antibodies in the blood of the woman is possible but is another test that has limited value. A woman's immune system can become exposed to a partner's sperm. For instance, this may be due to abrasions in the vagina during intercourse, and it has also been proposed to occur following oral or anal intercourse. When antisperm antibodies are found in the woman's blood there isn't a treatment that has been shown to be useful to suppress the antibodies. Once again, some women with a high level of the antibodies won't have a problem with fertility, and the level of antibodies provides limited, if any, predictive value about future success at becoming pregnant. It is another test result that is difficult to interpret, often creates anxiety, and rarely changes clinical management.

WHAT OPTIONS WILL I HAVE?

I usually suggest the couple return to my office after all the basic testing has been completed. That way we can review the test results together and discuss what options are available. If the testing reveals a specific problem the discussion is usually straightforward, centering on how to correct or compensate for the problem. If the testing is normal, the discussion will involve whether to start empiric treatment, or to consider other testing, such as a laparoscopy.

When to perform a diagnostic laparoscopy is debatable. Your own personal medical history is often the best indicator of when a diagnostic laparoscopy should be performed. Laparoscopy is necessary to visualize and treat pelvic endometriosis and scar tissue. In most cases, other imaging techniques, such as ultrasound, hysterosalpingogram, MRI, and CT cannot visualize either endometriosis or scarring, referred to as adhesions. If any or all of these other tests are normal, it does not rule out endometriosis or pelvic adhesive disease. A physical exam is also a poor screening test for endometriosis. Sometimes implants of endometriosis can be palpated on a pelvic or rectal exam, but more often they are not able to be felt.

Endometriosis is a disease when the lining of the uterus,

called the endometrium, implants outside the uterine cavity. The implants are usually found inside the pelvic cavity and cause inflammation (and ultimately scar tissue) that can reduce fertility, create significant pain especially around the time of menstrual bleeding, and may lead to uncomfortable intercourse. It affects about 50 percent of women with excessively painful menstrual periods and about 25 percent of subfertile women.

The Endometriosis Association (*www.endometriosisassn .org*) is an excellent resource for learning about this problem in more detail. Most experts agree that removing the endometriosis improves fertility. A study in 1997 by Dr. Macoux and colleagues published in the *New England Journal of Medicine* showed that even women with minimal or mild endometriosis received a fertility benefit from surgical removal of the endometriosis. It is clear that surgical removal of endometriosis can also reduce both menstrual period pain and painful intercourse.

Strictly speaking, a laparoscopy is necessary to rule out adhesions as the cause of infertility. Scar tissue may not actually be blocking the Fallopian tubes but it can still cause infertility. Scar tissue around the ovaries can prevent the egg from reaching the Fallopian tube. Scarring around the Fallopian tube(s) can also have the same result, keeping the sperm and egg from uniting. Removing the scar tissue at the time of laparoscopy is recommended but not always successful. Keep in mind that scar tissue can re-form in the process of healing following the surgery. You may have noticed that some people develop a great deal of scar tissue in the healing process, whereas with others you can hardly see the scar. Well-trained pelvic surgeons use special techniques to promote good healing and minimize scar tissue formation, but despite the best surgical technique, it is often unsuccessful.

Figure 12.3

REASONS TO CONSIDER A DIAGNOSTIC LAPAROSCOPY

- Painful menstrual periods
- Unexplained infertility
- Painful intercourse
- History of a pelvic infection, such as pelvic inflammatory disease (PID)
- History of a ruptured appendix
- Previous pelvic surgery
- Failed medical therapy
- Prolonged infertility
- Advanced maternal age

WHAT IF A CAUSE CANNOT BE FOUND?

Once all testing is completed, often the cause of the infertility is "unexplained." It is frustrating and unsatisfying to both the couple and the doctor, because the problem that needs to be corrected isn't clear. I explain to couples who have this diagnosis that unfortunately we lack good tests for some of the problems that may lead to infertility. Of course, everyone wants to know what the cause is, but frequently we don't have an answer.

How can I prove that the egg is actually leaving the ovary at the time of ovulation, or that the sperm is capable of fertilizing the egg, or that the Fallopian tube can push a fertilized egg down into the uterus, or that a fertilized egg can implant in the uterus? In general I can't prove any of these things. I'm not saying there are no tests for these issues, but they are not considered clinically useful tests at the present time and are usually not recommended. For instance, a hamster egg penetration test used to be commonly applied to prove that a sperm could fertilize a hamster egg. This is no longer used because, although interesting, it only proves a man can or cannot fertilize a hamster egg and is not very predictive of success in fertilizing his wife's egg. This is a great example of a test that mostly creates only anxiety and is not clinically useful.

A word of caution: just because a test is available does not mean you should receive it. Until validated as clinically useful in large populations, a test is often a waste of your money, and a potential source of anxiety that often does not change clinical management. Be cautious of the practitioner who attempts to order every test available. If you have a concern about a test that is being ordered, ask the practitioner how the result of the test will influence your treatment. For the newer tests, and those not commercially available, your insurance company may not cover the cost. Often this will end up being a "wallet biopsy" more than anything else.

PUTTING YOUR TREATMENT IN PERSPECTIVE

When considering the best therapy for the unexplained infertile couple, the doctor should clearly explain all of the options. The doctor should then give a recommendation about which treatment he or she thinks is the best one for you. However, keep in mind that every couple is unique in so many ways. Infertility involves a complex interplay of medical, emotional, psychological, interpersonal, spiritual/religious, and financial issues. Given nearly identical medical circumstances I find that couples come to completely different conclusions about the treatment they prefer. Your physician should understand the complexity of the situation and be flexible in order to tailor the treatment to meet your specific needs. But you must be your own advocate and do your best to help your doctor understand all of your needs.

What is medically the "best" choice is frequently not the treatment that a couple chooses. If your physician is pushing you to do a treatment you don't feel comfortable with, you must *speak up*. You and your physician need to work together to formulate a treatment that best meets your needs.

What are some examples of this complexity? In Virginia, where I live, we have limited insurance coverage for medical or surgical treatment of infertility. Frequently, I explain to couples that a more expensive treatment is more likely to be successful, but due to financial limitations we take a more cost-effective approach initially, hoping to have some luck without needing to undergo the more expensive treatments. Another example is recommending intrauterine insemination (IUI) of sperm as a useful treatment. Some couples just aren't prepared to take the step of replacing sex with an office procedure. Other couples have specific religious concerns about IUI or in vitro fertilization (IVF) and choose other options, regardless of reduced success rates. The last example is the couple who is emotionally exhausted with the process and wants to move to the most likely treatment to become pregnant, often regardless of cost. This is almost always IVF these days.

As you are weighing your options, make sure you ask your doctor what the success rate is for a treatment and how it compares to the other options. The cost of each treatment is also important if insurance won't be covering it. Finding out how the success rates of different treatments compare to one another is key to understanding cost-effectiveness.

You don't have to decide while sitting in the office. Go home with the literature given to you by the doctor, search the Internet, and consider it further. Don't hesitate to make another appointment to talk with your doctor to ask other questions, and be clear before you move forward and make the decision best suited to your needs.

A Three-Month Pre-Pregnancy Planner

THREE MONTHS (OR GREATER)
PRIOR TO CONCEPTION CYCLE

- Make an appointment with your doctor for a preconceptional counseling visit.

At your preconceptional visit:

- Discuss immunizations/infections with your doctor.

Testing Strongly Recommended:
- Rubella/Varicella (Chicken Pox)—immunize three months prior to conceiving if you are not immune.
- Bacterial vaginosis—screening and treatment with antibiotics if infected.

Testing Suggested:
- HIV/Syphilis/Gonorrhea/Chlamydia
- Cystic Fibrosis carrier screening

Testing Offered If in a Risk Group:

- If in a risk group, testing can be offered for Toxoplasmosis/Tuberculosis/Cytomegalovirus
- Discuss all chronic medications or medical problems with your doctor. If your menstrual cycles are less than 23 days or greater than 35 days apart have this evaluated by your doctor.
- Have your doctor perform a physical exam.
- Discuss genetic counseling with your doctor or genetics counselor if you are 35 years of age or older or have a personal or family history of inheritable conditions.

Miscellaneous Considerations

- Both partners should stop smoking and avoid exposure to secondhand smoke.
- The male partner should stop drinking alcohol.
- The male partner should supplement his diet with a daily multivitamin that includes the RDA of vitamins and minerals. He should avoid megadosing with the exception of vitamin E, 300 milligrams twice a day. He should supplement with selenium and folate.
- Make plans well ahead of time to stop your birth-control method if you use the birth control pill, patch, or ring, Norplant, an IUD, Depo-Provera, or Implanon.
- Learn about your menstrual cycles by doing a BBT (basal-body-temperature) chart for one or two cycles.
- Avoid potentially harmful environmental exposures.
- Review details of your health insurance policy as it relates to pregnancy, labor, and postpartum care.
- Familiarize yourself with your company's maternity leave policy.

- Discuss with your partner the financial, professional, and personal changes that will take place after the baby is born.

If you are underweight and have short, irregular, or absent menstrual cycles:

- Gain at least the number of pounds that equals 5 percent of your ideal body weight. (For example, a six-pound weight gain for a woman who should weigh about 125 pounds.) If not successful, gain the number of pounds required to bring your body mass index (BMI) up to 20 (see Figure 6.1) and your body fat percentage above 22 percent (see Figure 6.2).
- Keep a menstrual calendar and note when ovulation occurs and menstrual bleeding begins to rule out luteal phase deficiency.

If you are overweight:

- If you have abnormal menstrual cycles, try to lose at least 5 percent of your weight, as it may improve fertility. Excessive weight is also associated with increased rates of miscarriage and pregnancy complications.

TWO MONTHS PRIOR TO CONCEPTION CYCLE

- Start taking a prenatal vitamin with 0.4 milligrams to 0.8 milligrams of folic acid, if you haven't already.

  If you had a previously affected child, or a parent, sibling, or other close relative was previously affected with a neural tube defect, discuss the correct dose of folic acid with your physician.

- Consider whether you exercise too much and make adjustments to your exercise habits.

  Keep in mind that excessive exercise can lead to decreased fertility and an increased risk of miscarriage.

ONE MONTH PRIOR TO CONCEPTION CYCLE

- Choose an ovulation-prediction method. I strongly recommend using home ovulation-prediction kits.
- The female partner should stop drinking alcohol and caffeinated beverages.
- If taking oral contraceptives up until the cycle of conception, increase dose of folic acid to 1.0 milligrams each day, beginning at least one month prior to conception.
- Do not take an aspirin a day to try to improve fertility.
- Consider additional iron supplementation if you have been previously diagnosed with iron-deficiency anemia.
- Assure dietary protein consumption of at least 60 to 75 grams per day.
- If you are a vegetarian, you need to be especially vigilant about potential nutritional deficiencies.

CONCEPTION CYCLE—YOUR PERSONALIZED CONCEPTION CALENDAR

Directions and Recommendations

A blank conception calendar can be found on page 294.

- Number your first day of menstrual bleeding in the space provided; label all subsequent cycle days.

- Indicate the day of the month in the box provided to further personalize your calendar.
- You should have an idea of when you will ovulate from previous cycles. Indicate on your calendar your anticipated day of ovulation by checking the circle next to Anticipated Ovulation.
- Five days prior to the anticipated ovulation, begin having intercourse every 36 to 48 hours. Check the circle next to Intercourse on the calendar on the appropriate days.
- If you are using an ovulation-prediction kit, refer to Figure 5.3 to determine what day to begin your daily urinary testing. Specify on your calendar the days to do your testing by checking the circle next to Urinary Testing. Remember that your daily urinary testing should be performed in the late morning for optimal results.
- Indicate on your calendar the day you ovulate by checking the circle next to Ovulation. Have intercourse the day of a positive result from your urinary ovulation-prediction testing and again 24 hours later.
- Do not use penile/vaginal lubricants.
- After intercourse the woman should lie on her back and elevate her hips for at least 15 to 30 minutes.

Sunday	Monday	Tuesday	Wednesday	Thursday	Friday	Saturday
Cycle day: _____ Date ___ ○ Anticipated Ovulation ○ Urinary Testing +/− ○ Intercourse ○ Ovulation ○ Cervical mucus: ___	Cycle day: _____ Date ___ ○ Anticipated Ovulation ○ Urinary Testing +/− ○ Intercourse ○ Ovulation ○ Cervical mucus: ___	Cycle day: _____ Date ___ ○ Anticipated Ovulation ○ Urinary Testing +/− ○ Intercourse ○ Ovulation ○ Cervical mucus: ___	Cycle day: _____ Date ___ ○ Anticipated Ovulation ○ Urinary Testing +/− ○ Intercourse ○ Ovulation ○ Cervical mucus: ___	Cycle day: _____ Date ___ ○ Anticipated Ovulation ○ Urinary Testing +/− ○ Intercourse ○ Ovulation ○ Cervical mucus: ___	Cycle day: _____ Date ___ ○ Anticipated Ovulation ○ Urinary Testing +/− ○ Intercourse ○ Ovulation ○ Cervical mucus: ___	Cycle day: _____ Date ___ ○ Anticipated Ovulation ○ Urinary Testing +/− ○ Intercourse ○ Ovulation ○ Cervical mucus: ___
Cycle day: _____ Date ___ ○ Anticipated Ovulation ○ Urinary Testing +/− ○ Intercourse ○ Ovulation ○ Cervical mucus: ___	Cycle day: _____ Date ___ ○ Anticipated Ovulation ○ Urinary Testing +/− ○ Intercourse ○ Ovulation ○ Cervical mucus: ___	Cycle day: _____ Date ___ ○ Anticipated Ovulation ○ Urinary Testing +/− ○ Intercourse ○ Ovulation ○ Cervical mucus: ___	Cycle day: _____ Date ___ ○ Anticipated Ovulation ○ Urinary Testing +/− ○ Intercourse ○ Ovulation ○ Cervical mucus: ___	Cycle day: _____ Date ___ ○ Anticipated Ovulation ○ Urinary Testing +/− ○ Intercourse ○ Ovulation ○ Cervical mucus: ___	Cycle day: _____ Date ___ ○ Anticipated Ovulation ○ Urinary Testing +/− ○ Intercourse ○ Ovulation ○ Cervical mucus: ___	Cycle day: _____ Date ___ ○ Anticipated Ovulation ○ Urinary Testing +/− ○ Intercourse ○ Ovulation ○ Cervical mucus: ___
Cycle day: _____ Date ___ ○ Anticipated Ovulation ○ Urinary Testing +/− ○ Intercourse ○ Ovulation ○ Cervical mucus: ___	Cycle day: _____ Date ___ ○ Anticipated Ovulation ○ Urinary Testing +/− ○ Intercourse ○ Ovulation ○ Cervical mucus: ___	Cycle day: _____ Date ___ ○ Anticipated Ovulation ○ Urinary Testing +/− ○ Intercourse ○ Ovulation ○ Cervical mucus: ___	Cycle day: _____ Date ___ ○ Anticipated Ovulation ○ Urinary Testing +/− ○ Intercourse ○ Ovulation ○ Cervical mucus: ___	Cycle day: _____ Date ___ ○ Anticipated Ovulation ○ Urinary Testing +/− ○ Intercourse ○ Ovulation ○ Cervical mucus: ___	Cycle day: _____ Date ___ ○ Anticipated Ovulation ○ Urinary Testing +/− ○ Intercourse ○ Ovulation ○ Cervical mucus: ___	Cycle day: _____ Date ___ ○ Anticipated Ovulation ○ Urinary Testing +/− ○ Intercourse ○ Ovulation ○ Cervical mucus: ___
Cycle day: _____ Date ___ ○ Anticipated Ovulation ○ Urinary Testing +/− ○ Intercourse ○ Ovulation ○ Cervical mucus: ___	Cycle day: _____ Date ___ ○ Anticipated Ovulation ○ Urinary Testing +/− ○ Intercourse ○ Ovulation ○ Cervical mucus: ___	Cycle day: _____ Date ___ ○ Anticipated Ovulation ○ Urinary Testing +/− ○ Intercourse ○ Ovulation ○ Cervical mucus: ___	Cycle day: _____ Date ___ ○ Anticipated Ovulation ○ Urinary Testing +/− ○ Intercourse ○ Ovulation ○ Cervical mucus: ___	Cycle day: _____ Date ___ ○ Anticipated Ovulation ○ Urinary Testing +/− ○ Intercourse ○ Ovulation ○ Cervical mucus: ___	Cycle day: _____ Date ___ ○ Anticipated Ovulation ○ Urinary Testing +/− ○ Intercourse ○ Ovulation ○ Cervical mucus: ___	Cycle day: _____ Date ___ ○ Anticipated Ovulation ○ Urinary Testing +/− ○ Intercourse ○ Ovulation ○ Cervical mucus: ___
Cycle day: _____ Date ___ ○ Anticipated Ovulation ○ Urinary Testing +/− ○ Intercourse ○ Ovulation ○ Cervical mucus: ___	Cycle day: _____ Date ___ ○ Anticipated Ovulation ○ Urinary Testing +/− ○ Intercourse ○ Ovulation ○ Cervical mucus: ___	Cycle day: _____ Date ___ ○ Anticipated Ovulation ○ Urinary Testing +/− ○ Intercourse ○ Ovulation ○ Cervical mucus: ___	Cycle day: _____ Date ___ ○ Anticipated Ovulation ○ Urinary Testing +/− ○ Intercourse ○ Ovulation ○ Cervical mucus: ___	Cycle day: _____ Date ___ ○ Anticipated Ovulation ○ Urinary Testing +/− ○ Intercourse ○ Ovulation ○ Cervical mucus: ___	Cycle day: _____ Date ___ ○ Anticipated Ovulation ○ Urinary Testing +/− ○ Intercourse ○ Ovulation ○ Cervical mucus: ___	Cycle day: _____ Date ___ ○ Anticipated Ovulation ○ Urinary Testing +/− ○ Intercourse ○ Ovulation ○ Cervical mucus: ___

Month:

Dietary Information for a
Sex-Selection Diet

Please refer to the Nutrition Section of Chapter 11 to understand how Appendix B can be used to assist you to create a sex-selection diet.

SUPPLEMENT INFORMATION

Potassium

- 99 milligrams per tablet
  GNC Potassium Gluconate 99
  Nature's Way Potassium
  TwinLab Minerals Potassium
- 500 milligrams per tablet
  Bromelain Hi Potassium
- 600 milligrams per tablet
  SlowK

Calcium

- Citrical*—630 milligrams Calcium and 400 IU of Vitamin D
- Caltrate**—600 milligrams Calcium and 400 IU of Vitamin D

- Tums**—500 milligrams Calcium
- Viactive**—500 milligrams Calcium

*Calcium source is calcium citrate and is the best absorbed supplement but contains less elemental (or absorbable) calcium, so more may need to be taken to meet the calcium requirement. Check the label to see milligrams of elemental calcium. Calcium citrate does not need to be taken with food to maximize absorption.

**Calcium source is calcium carbonate and is less readily absorbed but has more elemental calcium. Calcium carbonate needs to be taken with meals to maximize absorption.

Magnesium

- Magnesium Chelate—100 milligrams of magnesium and 47 milligrams of calcium per tablet
- Solgar Magnesium Glycinate—100 milligrams of magnesium per tablet
- SlowMag—114 milligrams of magnesium chloride and 106 milligrams of calcium per tablet
- Vitamin Shoppe Magnesium Chloride—62 milligrams of elemental magnesium per tablet

Nutrient Content of Breakfast Foods—Amounts Listed in Milligrams

Food	Magnesium	Calcium	Sodium	Potassium
Apple, large	11	13	2	227
Bagel, 4–5 oz	38	24	700	132
Banana, large	37	7	1	487
Bran flakes, ¾ cup	64	17	220	185
Canadian bacon, 2 oz	11	3	569	156
Cheerios, 1 cup	39	122	213	209
Cottage cheese, 2%, ½ cup	7	78	459	108
Cranberry juice, 1 cup (8 oz)	3	8	5	35
Cream of Wheat, instant, made with water, ½ cup	7	5	77	24
Egg substitute, liquid, ¼ cup	6	33	111	207
Egg whites, 1 large	4	2	55	54
Egg, 1 large	6	26	70	67
English muffin, whole	12	30	264	75
Frosted Flakes, ¾ cup	2	2	148	23
Grapefruit, large	13	20	0	231
Grits, quick, white, made with water, ½ cup	6	4	2	25
Milk, 2%, 1 cup	27	285	100	366
Milk, skim, 1 cup	27	306	103	382
Oatmeal, instant, made with water, 1 packet	38	110	78	105
Orange juice, 1 cup (8 oz)	27	25	2	473
Orange, large	18	74	0	333
Sausage, 1 link	4	4	201	57
Shredded Wheat, 1 cup	57	21	3	203
Turkey bacon, 1 oz, cooked	5	1	366	63
Wheat bread, 1 slice	12	26	132	50
White bread, 1 slice	7	45	204	30
Yogurt, light, 8 oz	0	216	102	331
Yogurt, low-fat, fruit, 8 oz	30	313	120	402

Nutrient Content of Lunch Foods—Amounts Listed in Milligrams

Food	Magnesium	Calcium	Sodium	Potassium
Cheddar cheese, 1 oz	8	202	174	27
Cheddar cheese, low-sodium, 1 oz	6	197	6	31
Ham, deli style, 2 oz	20	6	849	178
Ham, cured, low-sodium, 2 oz	9	5	640	189
Jams and preserves, 1 Tbsp	1	4	6	15
Mozzarella cheese, part-skim, 1 oz	7	222	175	24
Mozzarella cheese, part-skim, low-sodium, 1 oz	7	222	4	27
Muenster cheese, 1 oz	8	201	176	38
Pasteurized process American cheese, 1 oz	8	155	417	47
Pasteurized process American cheese, low-sodium, 1 oz	9	129	359	1
Peanut butter, creamy, 2 Tbsp	49	14	147	208
Peanut butter, no salt added, creamy, 2 Tbsp	49	14	5	208
Pita, whole wheat, 6½ inch	44	10	340	109
Provolone cheese, 1 oz	8	212	245	39
Ricotta cheese, part skim, ½ cup	19	337	155	155
Roast beef, thin sliced, deli-style, 2 oz	12	6	906	270
Salad, fruit, canned in water, 1 cup	12	17	7	191
Salad, vegetables, no dressing, 1½ cups	23	27	54	356
Swiss cheese, 1 oz	11	221	54	22
Swiss cheese, low-sodium, 1 oz	10	269	4	31
Tortilla, flour, 8 inch	0	97	249	0
Tuna, light, canned in water, 3 oz	23	9	287	201
Tuna, light, canned in water, without salt, 3 oz	23	9	42	201
Turkey, deli style, oven roasted, 2 oz	15	6	668	115
Wheat bread, 1 slice	12	132	132	50
White bread, 1 slice	7	204	204	25

Nutrient Content of Dinner Foods—Amounts Listed in Milligrams

Food	Magnesium	Calcium	Sodium	Potassium
Artichokes (hearts), cooked, ½ cup	50	38	80	297
Beef, pot roast, cooked, 3 oz	16	14	40	196
Beef, sirloin, cooked, 3 oz	19	8	48	281
Black Beans, ½ cup	60	23	204	305
Broccoli, cooked, 1 cup	33	62	64	457
Chicken Vegetable Soup, ready-to-serve, 1 cup	10	26	1068	367
Chicken, skinless, boneless, cooked, 3 oz	29	15	74	256
Corn, cooked, 1 large ear	38	2	299	294
Green beans, cooked, 1 cup	22	55	1	182
Ground Beef, 10% fat, cooked, 3 oz	23	14	74	368
Ground Turkey, 10% fat, cooked, 3 oz	20	20	88	221
Haddock, cooked, 3 oz	42	36	74	399
Halibut, cooked, 3 oz	91	51	59	490
Kidney Beans, ½ cup	34	44	303	379
Marinara sauce, ready to serve, ½ cup	26	34	601	470
Pork chop, center loin, cooked, 3 oz	15	22	50	300
Potato, baked, 1 medium	48	26	17	926
Rice, brown, cooked, ½ cup	42	10	5	42
Rice, white, instant, cooked, ½ cup	7	10	5	13
Salmon, cooked, 3 oz	26	13	52	326
Snap peas, cooked, 1 cup	42	67	6	384
Spaghetti, enriched, cooked, 1 cup	25	10	1	53
Spaghetti, whole wheat, cooked, 1 cup	42	21	4	62
Spinach, cooked from fresh, 1 cup	157	245	126	839
Sweet potato, 1 medium	31	43	41	542
Tofu, firm, prepared with nigaria , ½ cup	48	159	7	120
Tuna, yellowfin, cooked, 3 oz	54	14	41	377
Turkey, dark meat, cooked, 3 oz	24	32	79	290
Turkey, light meat, cooked, 3 oz	28	19	64	305
Vegetable Soup, ready-to-serve, 1 cup	7	55	1010	396

Nutrient Content of Snack Foods—Amounts Listed in Milligrams

Food	Magnesium	Calcium	Sodium	Potassium
Almonds, dry roast, no salt added, 1 oz	81	75	0	211
Almonds, dry roast, salt added, 1 oz	81	75	96	211
Cashews, dry roasted, no salt added, 1 oz	74	13	5	160
Cashews, dry roasted, salt added, 1 oz	74	13	181	160
Graham crackers, plain or honey, 1 sheet	4	3	85	19
Granola bar, hard plain, 1 bar	25	15	74	84
Granola bar, soft, chocolate chip, 1 bar	34	40	117	176
Honeydew melon, 1/8 medium	12	8	2	285
Peach, large	14	9	0	198
Peanuts, dry roasted, no salt added, 1 oz	50	15	2	187
Peanuts, dry roasted, salt added, 1 oz	50	15	230	187
Popcorn, air popped, 3 cups	35	2	2	79
Popcorn, low fat, low salt, microwave, 3 cups	38	3	122	60
Potato chips, plain, 1 oz	20	7	149	466
Potato chips, plain, unsalted, 1 oz	19	7	2	361
Pretzels, hard, salted, 10 twists	17	11	814	88
Pudding, chocolate, ready made, 4 oz	24	102	146	203
Salsa	10	18	396	196
Snack crackers, saltines, low-fat, low salt, 6	8	7	191	34
Strawberries, 1 cup sliced	22	27	2	254
Tortilla chips, plain, white corn, 1 oz	41	49	119	61
Tortilla chips, plain, white corn, unsalted, 1 oz	38	45	56	52

GLOSSARY

amniocentesis: A procedure in which an ultrasound-guided needle takes a small amount of fluid from the sac of amniotic fluid around a baby, later to be used for chromosome analysis.

bacterial vaginosis: An overgrowth of bacteria in the vagina, resulting in excessive discharge that is commonly "milky" in appearance and "fishy" in smell; associated with preterm labor and late miscarriage.

chorionic villus sampling: A procedure performed during the late first trimester of pregnancy in which small pieces of the placenta are removed for chromosome analysis.

chromosomes: Microscopic structures found in nearly all living cells, containing the DNA codes that tell the body how to make up each unique individual.

congenital disorder: A disease or condition that affects a baby prior to birth.

corpus luteum: The ovarian cyst that forms after ovulation and is responsible for production of progesterone during the luteal phase.

deoxyribonucleic acid (DNA): The basic building block of chromosomes, making up the fundamental genetic material in our body.

Down's syndrome: A genetic disorder caused by the presence of an extra twenty-first chromosome; also referred to as Trisomy 21.

Characterized by mental retardation (of varying severity), abnormal facial features and growth, and various other problems such as heart defects.

ectopic pregnancy: An abnormal pregnancy that occurs outside of the uterus, most commonly in a Fallopian tube.

embryo: The stage of the early pregnancy around the time when the fertilized egg implants in the lining of the uterus and begins to grow.

endometriosis: A disorder in which tissue similar to the lining of the uterus (the endometrium) implants and grows outside the uterine cavity. Often associated with severely painful menstrual periods and infertility.

endometrium: The lining of the uterus where the early embryo implants and grows.

estrogen: Often referred to as "the female hormone." Made by the ovary and responsible for the growth of the endometrium during the first half of the menstrual cycle.

fibroids: Common benign growths of smooth muscle in the uterus; most often without symptoms, but can enlarge uterine size, increase menstrual bleeding and cramping, and cause infertility or miscarriage.

follicle: A small cystic structure found in the ovaries; contains an egg inside.

follicle stimulating hormone (FSH): In a female, the hormone released by the pituitary gland during each cycle; responsible for stimulating the growth and maturation of a follicle containing an egg.

follicular phase: The period of time during the menstrual cycle that begins with the onset of menstrual bleeding and ends with the mid-cycle rise in lutenizing hormone.

gene: A sequence of DNA that codes for a specific trait or product made in the body. It is the basic unit of heredity.

human chorionic gonadotropin (hCG): The hormone produced during pregnancy; used for all forms of pregnancy testing.

infertility: A condition in which a couple is unable to get pregnant after one year of attempting to conceive.

insulin: A hormone secreted by the pancreas; chiefly responsible for regulating glucose (sugar) levels in the body.

in vitro fertilization (IVF): The process of collecting eggs from a woman and fertilizing them in a laboratory (also referred to as a "test-tube baby"). A certain number of the resulting embryos are then placed back into the uterus of the mother or a surrogate.

laparoscopy: A surgical procedure in which a camera mounted on a thin metal tube is inserted through the abdominal wall (usually under the navel) to visualize and operate on organs in the pelvis or abdomen.

luteal phase: The period of time during the menstrual cycle that begins with the rise of LH and ends with the onset of menstrual bleeding.

luteinizing hormone (LH): The hormone released from the pituitary gland that is responsible for release of the egg from the ovary, or ovulation; used to test for ovulation by home ovulation-prediction kits.

miscarriage: The spontaneous loss of a pregnancy prior to the time the fetus would be able to survive on its own outside of the mother.

neural tube defect: A birth defect involving the brain or spinal cord.

ovulation: Release of the egg from an ovarian follicle in response to a rise in luteinizing hormone (LH).

pituitary gland: A gland that lies adjacent to the brain and secretes hormones (such as LH and FSH) involved in many important bodily functions, including reproduction.

polycystic ovarian syndrome (PCOS): A common endocrinologic disorder associated with irregular or absent menstrual periods, excessive acne or unwanted hair growth, reduced fertility, and, usually, excessive weight.

progesterone: A hormone produced by women in the second half of the menstrual cycle; responsible for preparing the uterine lining for implantation of an embryo and supporting the growth of early pregnancy.

reproductive endocrinologist: A specially trained obstetrician/gynecologist for infertile couples, who deals with hormonal problems of women, and various other abnormalities of the female reproductive system.

teratogen: Any substance that can cause a birth defect when a woman is exposed to it before or during pregnancy.

RESOURCES

GENERAL INFORMATION ABOUT REPRODUCTIVE HEALTH

To do on-line searches of the medical literature and the complementary and alternative-medicine literature go to the National Library of Medicine at *www.igm.nlm.nih.gov*. Access to many of the premier U.S. university and medical center library systems: *www.healthweb.org*.

American College of Obstetricians and Gynecologists
409 12th Street, S.W.
Washington, D.C. 20024-2188
(202) 638-5577
www.acog.org

American Society of Reproductive Medicine
1209 Montgomery Highway
Birmingham, AL 35216-2809
(205) 978-5000
www.asrm.org

Endometriosis Association
www.endometriosisassn.org

Society for Reproductive Endocrinology and Infertility
www.srei.org

BIRTH DEFECTS

National Network to Prevent Birth Defects
Box 15309 S.E. Station
Washington, D.C. 20003
(202) 543-5450

March of Dimes
P.O. Box 1657
Wilkes-Barre, PA 18703
888-MODIMES
www.modimes.org

INFERTILITY SUPPORT

RESOLVE (Infertility Support Group and Resource)
5 Water Street
Arlington, MA 02174
(800) 662-1016
www.resolve.org

RESOURCES FOR QUESTIONS ABOUT EXPOSURE TO CHEMICALS IN
EARLY PREGNANCY (TERATOGENS)

If you live east of the Mississippi:
    Massachusetts Teratogen Information Service
    Boston, Massachusetts
    (617) 466-8474

If you live west of the Mississippi:
    Pregnancy Riskline
    Salt Lake City, Utah
    (801) 328-2229

Grateful Med (Toxline, Toxnet and Medline)
    (800) 638-8480
    *Access through the National Institutes of Health website at: *www*
    .nih.gov or through the National Library of Medicine at: *www.igm*
    .nlm.nih.gov

Reprotox
(202) 293-5137 (Washington, D.C.)

Reprorisk
(800) 525-9083
Shepherd's Catalog of Teratogenic Agents
(206) 543-3373 (Seattle, WA)

PRECONCEPTIONAL CARE

Robert C. Cefalo and Merry K. Moos, *Preconceptional Health Care: A Practical Guide,* 2nd ed., 1995, Mosby-Year Book, ISBN: 0815116381.

SELECTED READINGS

CHAPTER 1: THE BASICS

American College of Obstetricians and Gynecologists. *Planning for Pregnancy, Birth and Beyond.* 2d ed. Washington, D.C.: ACOG, 1995.

Wilcox, A. J., C. R. Weinberg, and D. D. Baird. "Timing of sexual intercourse in relation to ovulation: Effects on the probability of conception, survival of the pregnancy and the sex of the baby." *New England Journal of Medicine* 333, no. 23 (1995): 1519.

CHAPTER 2: AM I FERTILE?

Hay, P. E., R. F. Lamont, D. Taylor-Robinson, D. J. Morgan, C. Ison, and J. Pearson. "Abnormal bacterial colonisation of the genital tract and subsequent preterm delivery and late miscarriage." *British Medical Journal* 308, no. 6924 (1994): 295–98.

Llahi-Camp, J. M., R. Rai, C. Ison, L. Regan, and D. Taylor-Robinson. "Association of bacterial vaginosis with a history of second trimester miscarriage." *Human Reproduction* 11, no. 7 (1996): 1575–78.

Ralph, S. G., A. J. Rutherford, and J. D. Wilson. "Influence of bacterial vaginosis on conception and miscarriage in the first trimester:

cohort study." *British Medical Journal* 319, no. 7204 (1999): 220–23.

Weström, L. "Incidence, prevalence, and trends of acute pelvic inflammatory disease and its consequences in industrialized countries." *American Journal of Obstetrics and Gynecology* 138 (1980): 880.

CHAPTER 3: PRECONCEPTIONAL CARE

American College of Obstetricians and Gynecologists. "Preconceptual Care." *ACOG Technical Bulletin* 205. Washington, D.C.: ACOG, 1995.

American College of Obstetricians and Gynecologists. "Rubella and pregnancy." *ACOG Technical Bulletin* 171. Washington, D.C.: ACOG, 1992.

American College of Obstetricians and Gynecologists. "Teratology." *ACOG Technical Bulletin* 84. Washington, D.C.: ACOG, 1985.

American College of Obstetricians and Gynecologists. "Vitamin A supplementation during pregnancy." ACOG Committee Opinion 196. Washington, D.C.: ACOG, 1995.

Callahan, T. L., et al. "The economic impact of multiple-gestation pregnancies and the contribution of assisted-reproductive techniques to their incidence." *New England Journal of Medicine* 331, no. 4 (1994): 244–49.

Cefalo, R. C., W. A. Bowes, Jr., and M-K Moos. "Preconception care: a means of prevention." *Bailliere's Clinical Obstetrics and Gynaecology* 9, no. 3 (1995): 403–430.

Centers for Disease Control and Prevention. "Knowledge and use of folic acid by women of childbearing age—United States, 1997." *JAMA: Journal of the American Medical Association* 278, no. 11 (1997): 892–93.

Centers for Disease Control and Prevention. "Recommendations for the use of folic acid to reduce the number of cases of spina bifida and other neural tube defects." *MMWR* 41, RR-14 (1992).

Dokken, B., and D. Johnson. "The importance of reaching preconception targets for glycemic control in diabetic women." *Archives of Internal Medicine* 158, no. 12 (1998): 1299–1300.

Hogge, J. S., and W. A. Hogge. "Preconception genetic counseling." *Clinical Obstetrics and Gynecology* 39, no. 4 (1996): 751–62.

Jensen, T. K., N. H. I. Hjollund, T. B. Henriksen, T. Scheike, H. Kolstad, A. Giwercman, E. Ernst, J. P. Bonde, N. E. Skakkebaek, and J. Olsen. "Does moderate alcohol consumption affect fertility? Follow-up study among couples planning first pregnancy." *British Medical Journal* 317, no. 7157 (1998): 505–510.

Kuter, B. J., R. E. Weibel, H. A. Guess, H. Matthews, D. H. Morton, and P. J. Neff, et al. "Oka/Merck varicella vaccine in healthy children: Final report of a 2-year efficacy study and 7-year follow-up studies." *Vaccine* 9 (1991): 643–47.

MRC Vitamin Study Research Group. "Prevention of neural tube defects: results of the MRC vitamin study." *Lancet* 338 (1991): 132–37.

Mushinski, M. "Average charges for uncomplicated vaginal, cesarean, and vbac deliveries: regional variations, United States, 1996." *Statistical Bulletin* (July–September 1998): 17–28.

Perlow, J. H. "Education about folic acid: the ob-gyn's role in preventing neural tube defects." *Contemporary Ob/Gyn* (March 1999): 39–53.

Zavos, P. M., and P. N. Zarmakoupis-Zavos. "How smoking affects reproductive health: Female fecundity." *OBG Management* (February 1999): 48–55.

CHAPTER 4: STOPPING BIRTH CONTROL

American College of Obstetricians and Gynecologists. "Contraceptives and congenital anomalies." ACOG Committee Opinion 124. Washington, D.C.: ACOG, 1993.

Bracken, M. B., K. G. Hellenbrand, and T. R. Holford. "Conception delay after oral contraceptive use: the effect of estrogen dose." *Fertility and Sterility* 53 (1990): 21–27.

Harlap, S., and M. Baras. "Conception-waits in fertile women after stopping oral contraceptives." *International Journal of Fertility* 29 (1984): 73–80.

CHAPTER 5: TIMING IS EVERYTHING: PREDICTING OVULATION

Bauman, J. "Basal body temperature: unreliable method of ovulation detection." *Fertility and Sterility* 36 (1982): 729–33.

Miller, P. B., and M. R. Soules. "The usefulness of a urinary LH kit for ovulation prediction during menstrual cycles of normal women." *Fertility and Sterility* 87 (1996): 13–17.

Quagliarello, J., and M. Arny. "Inaccuracy of basal body temperature charts in predicting urinary luteinizing hormone surges." *Fertility and Sterility* 45 (1986): 334–37.

CHAPTER 6: WEIGHT AND EXERCISE

Bullen, B. A., G. S. Skrinar, and I. Z. Beitins, et al. "Induction of menstrual disorders by strenuous exercise in untrained women." *New England Journal of Medicine* 312 (1985): 1349–53.

Clark, A. M., B. Thornley, L. Tomlinson, C. Galletley, and R. J. Norman. "Weight loss in obese infertile women results in improvement in reproductive outcome for all forms of fertility treatment." *Human Reproduction* 13, no. 6 (1998): 1502–5.

Flegal, K. M. (Centers for Disease Control and Prevention). "Trends in body weight and overweight in the U.S. population." *Nutrition Reviews* 54, no. 4, part 2 (1996): S97–100.

Frisch, R. E. "Body fat, menarche, fitness and fertility." *Human Reproduction* 2, no. 6 (1987): 521–33.

Green, B. B., N. S. Weiss, and J. R. Daling. "Risk of ovulatory infertility in relation to body weight." *Fertility and Sterility* 50 (1988): 721–26.

Grodstein, F., M. B. Goldman, and D. W. Cramer. "Body mass index and ovulatory infertility." *Epidemiology* 5, no. 2 (1994): 247–50.

Hogdgon, J. A., and M. B. Beckett. "Prediction of Percent Body Fat for U.S. Navy Women from Body Circumferences and Height." *Naval Health Research Center Report* No. 84–29. San Diego, California.

Institute of Medicine. Subcommittee for a Clinical Application Guide, Committee on Nutritional Status During Pregnancy and Lactation, Food and Nutrition Board, and the National Academy of Sciences. "Body mass index chart; nutrition during pregnancy and lactation." Washington, D.C.: National Academy Press, 1992.

Kuczmarski, R. J., M. D. Carroll, K. M. Flegal, and R. P. Trojano (Centers for Disease Control and Prevention). "Varying body mass index cutoff points to describe overweight prevalence among U.S. adults: NHANES III (1988 to 1994)." *Obesity Research* 5, no. 6 (1997): 542–48.

Norman, R. J., and A. M. Clark. "Obesity and reproductive disorders: a review." *Reproduction, Fertility, & Development* 10, no. 1 (1998): 55–63.

Serdula, M. K., A. H. Mokdad, D. F. Williamson, D. A. Galuska, J. M. Mendlein, and G. W. Heath. "Prevalence of attempting weight loss and strategies for controlling weight." *JAMA: Journal of the American Medical Association* 282, no. 14 (1999): 1353–58.

Speroff, L., R. H. Glass, and N. G. Kase. *Clinical Gynecologic Endocrinology and Infertility*, Sixth Edition. Lippincott, Williams & Wilkins, 1999, pp. 781–808.

Stein, J. "The Low-Carb Diet Craze." *Time* (November 1, 1999): 72–79.

CHAPTER 7: DIET AND NUTRITION

Chiaffarino, F., F. Parazzini, C. La Vecchia, L. Chatenoud, and E. Di Cintio. "Diet and uterine myomas." *Obstetrics and Gynecology* 94, no. 3 (1999): 395–98.

Check, J. H., C. Dietterich, D. Lurie, A. Nazari, and J. Chuong. "A matched study to determine whether low-dose aspirin without heparin improves pregnancy rates following frozen embryo transfer and/or affects endometrial sonographic parameters." *Journal of Assisted Reproductive Genetics* 15, no. 10 (1998): 579–82.

Covens, A. L., P. Christopher, and R. F. Casper. "The effect of dietary supplementation with fish oil fatty acids on surgically induced endometriosis in the rabbit." *Fertility and Sterility* 49, no. 4 (1988): 698–703.

Hakim, R. B., R. H. Gray, and H. Zacur "Alcohol and caffeine consumption and decreased fertility." *Fertility and Sterility* 78 (1998): 632–37.

Institute of Medicine. Subcommittee for a Clinical Application Guide, Committee on Nutritional Status During Pregnancy and Lactation, Food and Nutrition Board, and the National Academy of Sciences. "Dietary reference intakes. Nutrition during pregnancy and lactation." Washington, D.C.: National Academy Press, 1992.

Nestler, J. E., D. J. Jakubowicz, P. Reamer, R. D. Gunn, and A. Geoffrey. "Ovulatory and metabolic effects of d-chiro-inositol in the polycystic ovary syndrome." *New England Journal of Medicine* 340, no. 17 (1999): 1314–20.

Rubinstein, M., A. Marazzi, and E. Polak de Fried. "Low-dose aspirin treatment improves ovarian responsiveness, uterine and ovarian blood flow velocity, implantation, and pregnancy rates in patients undergoing in vitro fertilization: a prospective, randomized, double-blind placebo-controlled assay." *Fertility and Sterility* 71, no. 5 (1999): 825–29.

Torfs, C. P., E. A. Katz, T. F. Bateson, P. K. Lam, and C. J. Curry. "Maternal medications and environmental exposures as risk factors for gastroschisis." *Teratology* 54, no. 2 (1996): 84–92.

CHAPTER 8: THE MAN'S ROLE IN GETTING PREGNANT QUICKLY

Clarke, R. N., S. C. Klock, A. Geoghegan, and D. E. Travassos. "Relationship between psychological stress and semen quality among in-vitro fertilization patients." *Human Reproduction* 14, no. 3 (1999): 753–58.

Feichtinger, W. "Environmental factors and fertility." *Human Reproduction* 6, no. 8 (1991): 1170–75.

Figa-Talamanca, I., C. Cini, G. C. Varricchio, F. Dondero, L. Gandini, A. Lenzi, F. Lombardo, L. Angelucci, R. Di Grezia, and F. R. Patacchioli. "Effects of prolonged autovehicle driving on male reproduction function: a study among taxi drivers." *American Journal of Industrial Medicine* 30, no. 6 (1996): 750–58.

Geva, E., G. Bartoov, N. Zabludovsky, J. B. Lessing, L. Lerner-Geva, and A. Amit. "The effect of antioxidant treatment on human spermatozoa and fertilization rate in an in vitro fertilization program." *Fertility and Sterility* 66, no. 3 (1996): 430–434.

Hughes, C. M., S. E. Lewis, V. J. McKelvey-Martin, and W. Thompson. "The effects of antioxidant supplementation during Percoll preparation on human sperm DNA integrity." *Human Reproduction* 13, no. 5 (1998): 1240–47.

Ji, B. T., X. O. Shu, M. S. Linet, W. Zheng, S. Wacholder, Y. T. Gao, D. M. Ying, and F. Jin. "Paternal cigarette smoking and the risk of childhood cancer among offspring of nonsmoking mothers." *Journal of the National Cancer Institute* 89, no. 3 (1997): 238–44.

Kessopoulou, E., H. J. Powers, K. K. Sharma, M. J. Pearson, J. M. Russell, I. D. Cooke, and C. L. R. Barratt. "A double-blind randomized placebo cross-over controlled trial using the antioxidant vitamin E to treat reactive oxygen species associated male infertility." *Fertility and Sterility* 64, no. 4 (1995): 825–31.

Lansac, J. "Delayed parenting. Is delayed childbearing a good thing?" *Human Reproduction* 10, no. 5 (1995): 1033–35.

Meacham, R. B., and M. J. Murray. "Reproductive function in the aging male." *Urologic Clinics of North America* 21, no. 3 (1994): 549–56.

Munkelwitz, R. Gilbert. "Are boxer shorts really better? A critical analysis of the role of underwear type in male subfertility." *Journal of Urology* 160, no. 4 (1998): 1329–33.

Nagourney, E. "In search of a way to bolster the sperm." *The New York Times* (Health and Fitness section) (June 8, 1999): D7.

Pacifici, R., I. Altieri, L. Gandini, A. Lenzi, S. Pichini, M. Rosa, P. Zuccaro, and F. Dondero. "Nicotine, cotinine, and trans-3-hydroxycotionine levels in seminal plasma of smokers: effects on semen parameters." *Therapeutic Drug Monitoring* 15, no. 5 (1993): 358–63.

Scott, R., A. MacPherson, R. W. Yates, B. Hussain, and J. Dixon. "The effect of oral selenium supplementation on human sperm motility." *British Journal of Urology* 82, no. 1 (1998): 76–80.

Vine, M. F., C-K J. Tse, P-Chuan Hu, and K. Y. Truong. "Cigarette smoking and semen quality." *Fertility and Sterility* 1996; 65(4): 835–42.

Vine, M. F. "Smoking and male reproduction." *International Journal of Andrology* 19, no. 6 (1996): 323–37.

Wang, C., V. McDonald, A. Leung, L. Superlano, N. Berman, L. Hull, and R. Swerdloff. "Effect of increased scrotal temperature on sperm production in normal men." *Fertility and Sterility* 68, no. 2 (1997): 334–39.

CHAPTER 9: SEX AND FERTILITY

Belanger, K., B. Leaderer, K. Hellenbrand, T. R. Holford, J. McSharry, M. E. Power, and M. B. Bracken. "Spontaneous abortion and exposure to electric blankets and heated water beds." *Epidemiology* 9, no. 1 (1998): 36–42.

Chacho, K. J., C. W. Hage, and S. Shulman. "The relationship between female sexual practices and the development of antisperm antibodies." *Fertility and Sterility* 56, no. 3 (1991): 461–64.

Cutler, W. B., G. Preti, G. R. Huggins, B. Erickson, and C. R. Garcia. "Sexual behavior frequency and biphasic ovulatory menstrual cycles." *Physiology & Behavior* 34, no. 5 (1985): 805–10.

Li, D. K., H. Checkokway, and B. A. Mueller. "Electric blanket use during pregnancy in relation to the risk of congenital urinary tract anomalies among women with a history of subfertility." *Epidemiology* 6, no. 5 (1995): 485–59.

Partonen, T. "Short note: Melatonin-dependent infertility." *Medical Hypotheses* 52, no. 3 (1999): 269–70.

Rojansky, N., A. Brzezinski, and J. G. Schenker. "Seasonality in human reproduction: an update." *Human Reproduction* 7, no. 6 (1992): 735–45.

Stumpf, W. E., and E. Denny. "Vitamin D (Soltriol), light, and reproduction." *American Journal of Obstetrics and Gynecology* 161, no. 5 (1989) 1375–84.

van Roijen, J. H., A. K. Slob, W. L. Gianotten, G. R. Dohle, A. T. Vreeburg, and R. F. Weber. "Sexual arousal and the quality of semen produced by masturbation." *Human Reproduction* 11, no. 1 (1996): 147–51.

Wilson, B. W., G. M. Lee, M. G. Yost, K. C. Davis, T. Heimbingner, and R. L. Buschbom. "Magnetic field characteristics of electric bed-heating devices." *Bioelectromagnetics* 17, no. 3 (1996): 174–79.

CHAPTER 10: TURNING BACK THE CLOCK: GETTING PREGNANT AT 35 AND OLDER

Adams, M. M., G. P. Oakley, Jr., and J. S. Marks. "Maternal age and births in the 1980s." *JAMA. Journal of the American Medical Association* 247, no. 4 (1982): 493–94.

American Society for Reproductive Medicine. *Guideline for Practice. Age Related Infertility.* ASRM, 1995.

American Society for Reproductive Medicine. *Infertility: An Overview; a guide for patients* (Patient Information Series). ASRM, 1995.

Bongaarts, J. "Infertility After Age 30: A False Alarm," Comments. *Family Planning Perspectives* 14, no. 2 (1982): 77.

Corson, S. L. "Achieving and maintaining pregnancy after age 40." *International Journal of Fertility & Women's Medicine* 43, no. 5: 249–56.

Fédération CECOS, D. Schwartz, and M. J. Mayaux. "Female fecundity as a function of age." *New England Journal of Medicine* 306, no. 7 (1982): 404–06.

Fonteyn, V. J., and N. B. Isada. "Nongenetic implications of child-bearing after age thirty-five." *Obstetrical and Gynecological Survey* 43, no. 12 (1988): 709–19.

Gilbert, W. M., T. S. Nesbitt, and B. Danielsen. "Childbearing beyond age 40: pregnancy outcome in 24,032 cases. *Obstetrics and Gynecology* 93, no. 1 (1999): 9–14.

Gindoff, P., et al. "Reproductive potential in older women." *Fertility and Sterility* 46 (1986): 989.

Green, B. B., N. S. Weiss, and J. R. Daling. "Risk of ovulatory infertility in relation to body weight." *Fertility and Sterility* 50 (1988): 723.

Nasseir, A., and J. A. Grifo. "Genetics, age, and infertility." *Maturitas* 30, no. 2 (1998): 189–92.

Sauer, M. M., R. J. Paulson, and R. A. Lobo. "Oocyte donation to women of advanced reproductive age: pregnancy results and obstetrical outcomes." *Human Reproduction* 11, no. 11 (1996): 2540–43.

Speroff, L. "The effect of aging on fertility." *Current Opinion in Obstetrics and Gynecology* 6 (1994): 115–20.

Torgerson, D. J., R. E. Thomas, and D. M. Reid. "Mother's and daughter's menopausal ages: is there a link?" *European Journal of Obstetrics, Gynecology, & Reproductive Biology* 74, no. 1 (1997): 63–66.

Virro, M. R., and A. B. Shewchuk. "Pregnancy outcome in 242 conceptions after artificial insemination with donor sperm and effects of maternal age on the prognosis for successful pregnancy." *American Journal of Obstetrics and Gynecology* 148, no. 5 (1984): 518–24.

CHAPTER 11: CHOOSING THE SEX OF YOUR BABY

American College of Obstetricians and Gynecologists. "Sex selection." *ACOG Committee Opinion* 177. Washington, D.C.: ACOG, 1996.

American Society for Reproductive Medicine Ethics Committee Statement. Chapter 23, Reimplantation Genetic Diagnosis. *Fertility and Sterility* 62, no. 5 (1994): 66S.

Belkin, L. "Getting the girl." *The New York Times Magazine*. The New York Times Company, July 25, 1999.

Fugger, E. F., S. H. Black, K. Keyvanfar, and J. D. Schulman. "Births of normal daughters after MicroSort sperm separation and intrauterine insemination, in-vitro fertilization, or intracytoplasmic sperm injection." *Human Reproduction* 13, no. 9 (1998): 2367–70.

Gray, R. "Natural family planning and sex selection: fact or fiction?" *American Journal of Obstetrics and Gynecology* 165, no. 6 (1991): 1982–84.

Hossain, A. M., S. Barik, B. Rizk, and I. H. Thorneycroft. "Preconceptual sex selection: past, present, and future." *Archives of Andrology* 40, no. 1 (1998): 3–14.

James, W. H. "Sex ratios following the use of the Ericsson method of sex selection, and following ICSI." *Human Reproduction* 2659–60. (Comment on: *Human Reproduction* 13, no. 1 [January 1998]: 146–49.)

Maconochie, N., and E. Roman. "Sex ratios: are there natural variations within the human population?" *British Journal of Obstetrics and Gynecology* 104, no. 9: 1050–53.

Muehleis, P. M., and S. Y. Long. "The effects of altering the pH of seminal fluid on the sex ratio of rabbit offspring." *Fertility and Sterility* 27, no. 12 (1976): 1438–45.

Reubinoff, B. E., and J. G. Schenker. "New advances in sex preselection." *Fertility and Sterility* 66, no. 3 (1996): 343–50.

Rosner, F. "The biblical and Talmudic secret for choosing one's baby's sex." *Israel Journal of Medical Sciences* 15, no. 9 (1979): 784–87.

Stolkowski, J., and J. Lorrain. "Preconceptional selection of fetal sex." *International Journal of Gyneaecology and Obstetrics* 18 (1980): 440–43.

Wilcox, A. J., C. R. Weinberg, and D. D. Baird. "Timing of sexual intercourse in relation to ovulation—Effects on the probability of conception, survival of the pregnancy and the sex of the baby." *New England Journal of Medicine* 333, no. 23 (1995): 1517–21.

Zarutskie, P. W., C. H. Muller, M. Magone, and M. R. Soules. "The clinical relevance of sex selection techniques." *Fertility and Sterility* 54, no. 5 (1990): 891–905.

CHAPTER 12: WHEN NATURE NEEDS A BOOST: WHAT TO EXPECT FROM A FERTILITY DOCTOR

Busacca, M., M. Vignali. Ovarian endometriosis: from pathogenesis to surgical treatment. *Current Opinion of Obstetrics and Gynecology* 2003; 15(4): 321–26.

Coutifaris, C., E. Meyers, D. Guzick, M., Diamond, S. Carson, R. Legro, P. McGovern, W. Schlaff, B. Carr, M. Steinkampf, S. Silva, D. Vogel, P. Leppert: NICHD National Cooperative Reproductive Medicine Network. Histological dating of timed endometrial biopsy tissue is not related to fertility status. *Fertility and Sterility* 82, no. 5 (2004): 1264–72.

Guzick, D., J. W. Overstreet, P. Factor-Livak, C. Brazil, S. Nakajima, C. Coutifaris, S. Carson, P. Cisneros, M. Steinkampf, J. Hill, Xu. Don, D. Vogel. "Sperm Morphology, Motility, and Concentration in Fertile and Infertile Men." *Fertility and Sterility,* 345 (2001): 1388–93.

Guzick, D. S., M. W. Sullivan, G. D. Adamson, M. I. Cedars, R. J. Falk, E. P. Peterson, et al. "Efficacy of treatment for unexplained infertility." *Fertility and Sterility* 70 (1998): 2007–13.

Lucidi, R. S., J. D. Pierce, S. K. Kavoussi, C. A. Witz. "Prior fertility in the male partner does not predict a normal semen analysis." *Fertility and Sterility* 84 (2005): 793–4.

Macoux S., R. Maheux, S. Berube, et al. Canadian Collaboration Group on Endometriosis. "Laparoscopic surgery in infertile women with minimal or mild endometriosis." *New England Journal of Medicine* 377 (1997): 212–22.

Rawson, J. M. Prevalence of endometriosis in asymptomatic women. *Journal of Reproductive Medicine* 37, no. 7 (1991): 513–15.

van Montfrans Joris M., Annemieke Hoek, Marcel H. A. van Hooff, Corry H. de Koning, Nino Tonch, Cornelis B. Lambalk. "Predictive value of basal follicle-stimulating hormone concentrations in a general subfertility population." *Fertility and Sterility* 74, no. 1 (2000): 97–103.

APPENDIX B

Bowes, Anna De Planter. *Bowes & Church's Food Values of Portions Commonly* Used. Ed. Jean Pennington. 16th ed. Philadelphia: J.B. Lippincott Company, 1994.

Dietary Guidelines for Americans. January 2005. Department of Health and Human Services and Department of Agriculture. 6 April 2006. <*http://www.healthierus.gov/dietaryguidelines/*>.

NHLBI Health Information Center. *The DASH Eating Plan*. 2nd ed. Bethesda: NIH Publications, 2003.

USDA National Nutrient Database for Standard Reference, release 18. 6 April 2006. <*http://www.nal.usda.gov/fnic/foodcomp/search/*>.

WEB RESOURCES FOR READERS

Selected High Sodium Foods . . . and Low Sodium Alternatives
http://www.ndif.org/na9.html
Nutrient Database for Standard Reference
http://www.nal.usda.gov/fnic/foodcomp/search
Dietary Guidelines for Americans—Appendix B: Food Sources of Selected Nutrients
http://www.health.gov/dietaryguidelines/dga2005/document/html/appendixB.htm

INDEX

Page numbers in *italics* refer to illustrations and charts.

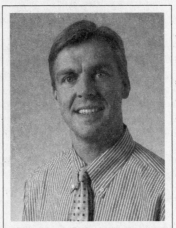

Photo by Tom Coghill, Courtesy of Martha Jefferson Hospital

ABOUT THE AUTHOR

Dr. Christopher Williams is the cofounder and director of the Reproductive Medicine and Surgery Center of Virginia, at Martha Jefferson Hospital, Charlottesville, Virginia. In addition to his busy clinical practice, Dr. Williams instructs resident physicians in Obstetrics and Gynecology from the University of Virginia and is involved in reproductive medicine and infertility research. He is a graduate of the University of Virginia School of Medicine. He completed his residency in Obstetrics and Gynecology at Carolinas Medical Center, in Charlotte, North Carolina, and underwent fellowship training in Reproductive Endocrinology and Infertility at the University of North Carolina at Chapel Hill. He is board certified in Obstetrics and Gynecology and subspecialty certified in Reproductive Endocrinology and Infertility. Dr. Williams lives in Charlottesville, Virginia, with his wife, Kara, their sons, Scott and Justin, and their daughter, Caroline.